Back Care

This book is to be returned on or before
the last date stamped below.

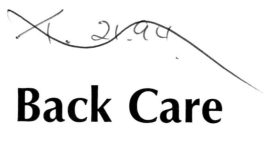

Back Care

An illustrated guide

Jean Oliver MCSP, SRP

Physiotherapist in Charge, Back Clinic, Cambridge;
Founder, Back Care Service; Director, Back Education Programme, Cambridge;
Postregistration Tutor for Physiotherapists.

Drawings by Ann Blythe

Anatomical illustrations by Jean Oliver

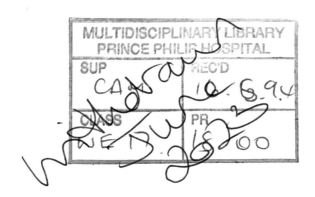
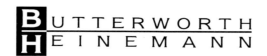

BUTTERWORTH
HEINEMANN

Butterworth-Heinemann Ltd
Linacre House, Jordan Hill, Oxford OX2 8DP

ℛ A member of the Reed Elsevier group

OXFORD   LONDON   BOSTON
MUNICH   NEW DELHI   SINGAPORE   SYDNEY
TOKYO   TORONTO   WELLINGTON

First published 1994

British Library Cataloguing in Publication Data
Oliver, Jean
  Back Care: Illustrated Guide
  I. Title   II. Blythe, Ann
  616.73

ISBN 0 7506 0191 4

Library of Congress Cataloguing in Publication Data
Oliver, Jean
  Back care: an illustrated guide/Jean Oliver; drawings by
  Ann Blythe; anatomical illustrations by Jean Oliver.
  p.   cm.
  Includes index.
  ISBN 0 7506 0191 4
  1. Backache – Atlases.   2. Back – Care and hygiene – Atlases.
  3. Backache – Exercise therapy – Atlases.   I. Title.
  [DNLM: 1. Back Pain – prevention & control – atlases.   2.Spine –
  physiology – atlases.   3. Back Pain – therapy – atlases.
  WE 17 04856]
  RD771.B217045
  617.5'64–dc20   93–6254
                                                           CIP

Typeset by TecSet Ltd, Wallington, Surrey
Printed and bound in Great Britain by
Martins the Printers,
Berwick-upon-Tweed

Contents

Preface   vii

Acknowledgements   ix

Introduction – General Principles   xi

1 Functional Anatomy   1
   The curves of the vertebral column   2
   Structure of a motion segment   4
   Movements of the spine   10
   Compression on the spine   12
   Pain   14

2 Syndromes   19
   Ligamentous syndromes   20
   Disc syndromes   26
   Facet syndrome   32
   Sacroiliac syndromes   38
   Syndromes related to structural faults   40
   Forward head syndrome   52

3 Posture   61
   Lying   62
   Sitting   76
   Standing   92

4 Lifting   107
   Leverage   108
   The individual's capacity for safe lifting   110
   General guidelines for lifting   112

5 Exercises   119
   General principles   122
   Exercises for pain relief   122
   Stretching and strengthening exercises   124
   Stretches for dysfunction   130
   Easing stiffness   130
   Exercises as part of a posture re-education programme   130
   Sport   130

6   Children and Teenagers   133
   Trauma   134
   Postural problems   134
   Seating   138
   Carrying   142
   Variations in ranges of movement   142
7   Pregnancy   145
   Causes of backache in pregnancy and postpartum   146
   Prevention   148

Index   158

Notes   162

Preface

Physiotherapists spend much of their time dealing with problems arising from spinal dysfunction. The number of working hours lost due to back pain is legion, yet even the high figures quoted underestimate the magnitude of the problem, since they often only include people earning a living, not housewives and young mothers. Economically disastrous though it may be for the country, for the patient chronic back pain can drive him to despair, ruining both job prospects and social relationships. Once a chronic lesion becomes established, it is increasingly difficult to manage. It therefore behoves everyone working in this field to consider how recurrences can be prevented and, even more importantly, how best we can employ ourselves in preventing lesions occurring in the first place.

The aim of this book is to help the therapist explain to the patient, by means of illustrations, how the spine functions, what may have gone wrong in his particular case, and how he can play an effective role in his own recovery and in the prevention of recurrences. The text on the left hand side of the book provides the background information for the therapist, pertaining to the illustrations. For simplicity only, throughout the text, the therapist is referred to as 'she' and the patient as 'he', but this is, of course, not necessarily the case in the drawings.

The use of mobilization and other modalities by the therapist may be necessary to restore full function, but if the root of the problem is misuse of the back, such treatment given *in isolation* is insufficient to prevent recurrence. Moreover, in the long term, it is inadvisable for the patient to rely solely on someone else manipulating his back to sort out his problem, while he continues to abuse it, albeit sometimes unknowingly. Without adequate muscular support, the motion segment is unstable, and good function can only be achieved in conjunction with the patient's own efforts. Some knowledge of functional anatomy and pathology will help to make the patient realize that the way he uses his back has an important influence on the healing process.

Establishing a link between what happens in the treatment session and how the patient uses his back for the rest of the time is essential, yet this link is often, surprisingly, absent. For example, there is little advantage in showing a patient backward pelvic tilting exercises to ease pain caused by repeated hyperextension if the patient continues to hyperextend his back during daily activities involving reaching, leaning, and so on.

All spinal conditions differ in some respects. Advice must, therefore, be specific to each patient. This often needs to be repeated at successive attendances: patients often forget what they have been told, especially at their first attendance, and some people are reluctant to ask questions for fear of appearing ignorant. When giving advice or an explanation, language appropriate to each patient should be used.

It is not easy for a patient to change his habitual way of life. All kinds of pressures may deter him: self-image, fixed attitudes, being over-worked, overtired, under mental stress, to name a few. If he thinks that too much is being asked of him, he will feel unable to comply and lose interest. It is more effective for the therapist to start with one aspect of back care that will be of particular value to the patient and, to begin with, concentrate on that. Once he is convinced of its effectiveness, the patient's interest is often stimulated so that he asks for guidance in other areas.

Therapists will be expected to act as role models and should be prepared to do so by having suitable chairs in the waiting area, etc. The approach used by each therapist will differ according to her particular personality and experience, but it should also take into account the patient's personality, circumstances and interests. If, for example, he is clearly not interested in performing exercises starting with advice on seating may be more acceptable to him. A positive approach, sense of humour, perseverance, and perhaps above all, being on equal terms with each patient will go a long way towards helping the patient to manage his back.

Acknowledgements

The motivation of many people over the years to manage their own back problems, not least that of my husband Peter, compelled me to write this book so that their experience could be used to the benefit of others. To illustrate the text, I was fortunate to be able to work with Ann Blythe, who took great care to produce both accurate and original drawings.

I would also like to thank the many chartered physiotherapists who have helped in different ways: Carmen Tarnowski who, many years ago, convinced me of the importance of good posture; Alison Middle-ditch and Jacky Balfour for their enthusiasm over the project and for their constructive reviews of the text; Jacquie Scott for her inspiration with regard to foot orthoses in relation to chronic back pain; Inge Newton of the Royal National Orthopaedic Hospital, London, for her elucidation of the Schroth method of treating scoliosis, also many of her staff including Helen Gray who checked my queries. In particular, I would like to express my gratitude to Margaret Polden and Jill Mantle for allowing me to make use of drawings in the chapter on Pregnancy from their excellent book, *Physiotherapy in Obstetrics and Gynaecology**. To merge with the style of this book, their illustrations, principally on pages 153 and 155, were redrawn. My thanks also to Jean Mould for giving her time to assist with this chapter.

I am indebted to Mike Adams, whose research is a continuing inspiration to all who are interested in biomechanics and the causes of back pain.

Finally, my grateful thanks go to Patricia Edwards for her assistance at very short notice with the typing of the manuscript and to Cambridge University Medical Library for allowing me to use their facilities.

*Polden M., Mantle J. (1990). *Physiotherapy in Obstetrics and Gynaecology*. Oxford: Butterworth-Heinemann.

To Peter and Elizabeth

Introduction –
General Principles

Before any advice is given to a patient concerning the care of his back, an assessment of his spinal condition by the physiotherapist is necessary to ascertain the degree of irritability of the lesion and to arrive at a clinical diagnosis.

It is a common misconception that the same advice applies to all patients. This cannot be so, given the variations in spinal structure, pathological conditions and degrees of irritability. Even minor structural variations influence where the line of gravity passes through the motion segment, governing the weight distribution through it. Advice must, therefore, be specific to each patient.

The spine has an amazing capacity quietly to store up microtrauma before pain is perceived. Although back pain may be triggered by a particular incident, usually one or more predisposing factors such as abnormal mechanics will have played a significant part. The more of these factors that are present, the more likely is the spine to yield under relatively little stress. Attention is often focused on the event which precipitated the attack of back pain, even though this may have simply been the 'last straw' following years of misuse — albeit unknowingly — of the back. Poor posture is the most common predisposing factor which insidiously renders the spine more vulnerable to additional mechanical stress and this is dealt with in detail in Chapter 3.

The patient's assessment should include a consideration of the following factors, which may reveal whether any predisposing causes have contributed to his problem.

1. Static versus dynamic muscle work

An insidious cause of symptoms, which is rarely apparent to patients, is the use of continuous static muscle work, e.g. in the back muscles of people using computers and in the neck muscles of musicians.

Static muscle work causes a rise of pressure within the muscles which compresses the blood vessels, decreasing the amount of blood flowing into them in proportion to the force of contraction (Grandjean, 1971). Waste products are not carried off and accumulate. This impairment of blood flow causes the muscles to fatigue, resulting in discomfort at first and, later, pain. At 60% of maximum force, the blood supply is stopped completely, and this can be endured for less than one minute. Lower forces can be endured for longer periods, but still have their limits and fatigue eventually occurs.

Dynamic muscle work, on the other hand, is far less fatiguing than static muscle work. When muscles work dynamically, contraction causes the blood to be expelled from them, followed by the relaxation phase, when a renewed flow of blood passes into the muscles. A good supply of sugar and oxygen, which are rich in energy, are brought to the muscles, and the removal of waste products is facilitated.

In occupations which incur the use of static muscle work, the affected muscles need to be both stretched and used dynamically at regular intervals to increase their circulation. Resting periodically may be insufficient to achieve this effect.

2. Range of movement

Many factors affect the range of movement possible at a joint. They include:

a. *Degree of ligamentous laxity*
    Using the 'average' degrees of movement in the population at large as a guide as to what a particular patient's range of movement

should be can be very misleading: many patients fall outside the norm and may be naturally hypo- or hypermobile, depending on their inherited degree of ligamentous laxity and bony structure. No amount of exercise will change a naturally hypomobile patient into a hypermobile one. The important consideration is what the patient's range of movement is at the present time compared with when he was in his late teens, taking into account his present age and pathological condition. A naturally hypermobile patient may experience symptoms with a small limitation of movement, though his existing full range of movement may well exceed that of a naturally hypomobile person.

b. *Age*
Although range of movement gradually diminishes after the age of 25, due to factors such as increasing disc stiffness, the patient's occupation and lifestyle also play an important part.

c. *Pathology*
Previous damage to the spine may have resulted in contracted scar tissue and loss of disc height. In the latter case, if disc narrowing is marked, full range of movement at that segmental level is neither possible nor desirable and, if forced, could lead to instability. Minor degenerative changes, however, do not necessarily affect range of movement.

To keep a healthy spine in good condition, its joints need to be taken through a full range of movement every day. Normal activities of daily living do not necessarily do this, but often participation in some sport restores a balance. Otherwise, a simple stretching regime is necessary. If, however, the spine is damaged in some way, the tissues should be stretched in accordance with the healing process and laying down of fibrous tissue. A stiff area in one part of the spine may have repercussions later by transferring stresses to adjacent segments. Too little or too much stretching both lead to dysfunction. All too often during the early healing process, the patient stresses the lesion too much, delaying the healing and leaving a weakened scar.

3. End of range positions
Joints do not normally like being held at the end of their range of movement for long periods. The structure that resists the end point of a particular movement responds by eventually becoming painful. An example is sitting for a sustained period with the knees in full extension without any support under them. When the position is finally released, the knees feel uncomfortable and are stiff to flex. The same occurs in the spine; a further example illustrates this. If a person with a very mobile spine sleeps in the prone position, the lumbar spine may initially not be in full extension, but if the spine stiffens, e.g. with increasing age, this position may then place it at the end of its extension range. Discomfort or pain is often then felt on rising due to sustained pressure on the apophyseal joints.

In upright postures, energy expenditure is reduced when people use their ligaments rather than muscles to maintain the postures. Hence people will stand with most weight on one leg, the hip pushed out to the side and the knee locked back into hyperextension, to avoid muscular fatigue. This soon becomes a habit and is responsible for many ligamentous strains in the hip, knee and back.

In a healthy spine, if a posture is to be held for a sustained period, somewhere in the region of the middle of the range is safer. In the lumbar spine, this would be midway between flexion and extension of a particular motion segment, with no rotation or lateral flexion to either side. This explains why the crook lying position is such a popular one when resting. Where pain and/or pathology are present, the middle of the range may be preferred, but often in the acute stage relief is obtained towards the end of the range of flexion or extension (*see* pp. 67–9). For a limited period of time, these near-end range positions may be usefully employed, but long term use can itself cause the kind of problems mentioned earlier.

4. Balance between activity and rest

In modern times, the concept of balance is unfashionable. Alexander in 1932 drew attention to the effect of body misuse, but many modern men and women pay lip service to this and continue to drive their bodies to the extreme, thinking they can get away with it. Few do, in fact, especially with the onset of middle age.

Caring for the spine is by no means always a question of curtailing people's activities. As far as possible, when the patient is ready, he should be encouraged to return to activities which he enjoys, but perhaps modify the way he does them. An incentive is that finding a painfree way of performing an activity often means that the patient can do it for longer than previously. Sedentary workers may need encouragement to use their spines more rather than less in order to improve circulation and nutrition to them.

The correct balance between activity and rest is individual to each person according to factors such as age, previous training and pathology. It is not always easy to achieve this due to pressures of living and unexpected duties such as caring for a sick relative. The physiotherapist can be invaluable in exploring with her patient how best he can find his correct measure.

References

Alexander F. M. (1932). *The Use of Self*. London: Methuen.
Grandjean E. (1971). *Fitting the Task to the Man. An Ergonomic Approach*. London: Taylor & Francis.

1
Functional Anatomy

In order to treat or give advice about any spinal condition, the physiotherapist must have an indepth knowledge of anatomy and biomechanics — and a summary is given below. For a more detailed account, *see* 'Further Reading'. The amount of detail required by different patients varies enormously; a short and simple explanation is all that some will require, while others will be interested in greater detail. The illustrations on the right hand pages provide this information. It is essential that language appropriate to each patient is used.

The Curves of the Vertebral Column
(Figs 1.1, 1.2)

Viewed from the side, the vertebral column ('backbone') is curved. *In utero*, the spine is in total flexion and, when reverse curves appear, they are termed 'secondary' curves. The first of these is in the neck, and it begins to develop during intrauterine life, accentuating when the baby starts to hold its head upright, forming the longer, lower cervical curve which extends from C2 to T2. In order for the head to be positioned so that the eyes see straight ahead, the upper cervical spine retains its primary curve. The lordotic curve in the lumbar region starts to form when the child begins to walk, but is not complete until he reaches 10 years of age (Kapandji, 1974). The remainder of the spine, i.e. thoracic and sacral regions, retain their primary, anterior concavities throughout life.

Viewed from the back, a slight lateral curve to the right or left is often seen in the upper thoracic spine, which may either be due to the dominance of one hand (i.e. in a right-handed individual the curve may be convex to the right, and *vice versa*) or to the position of the aorta.

The gentle curvatures depicted in Fig 1.1 enhance the shock absorbing capacity of the vertebral column. They help to dissipate forces applied to the spine so that the surrounding ligaments absorb some of them. In a significant number of people, however, one or more of the curves are either flattened, accentuated or out of alignment with the central axis of the body (*see* p. 95). Such spines are potentially at risk from mechanical stresses, but trauma only occurs if demands are made on the spine which are in excess of its capacity to withstand them. Flattened spines have a reduced capacity for shock absorption (Farfan, 1973) while, in a spine with an accentuated curve such as a hyperlordotic lumbar spine ('hollow back'), more stress is borne by the anterior longitudinal ligament and lower apophyseal joints, and problems of imbalance may arise, i.e. tightening and shortening of muscles and soft tissues spanning the concavity, with lengthening and weakening of tissues on the convex side. The degree to which each person is aware of, and respects, the capacities and limitations of his own spine will have an important influence on the health or state of degeneration of it.

Curves of the spine

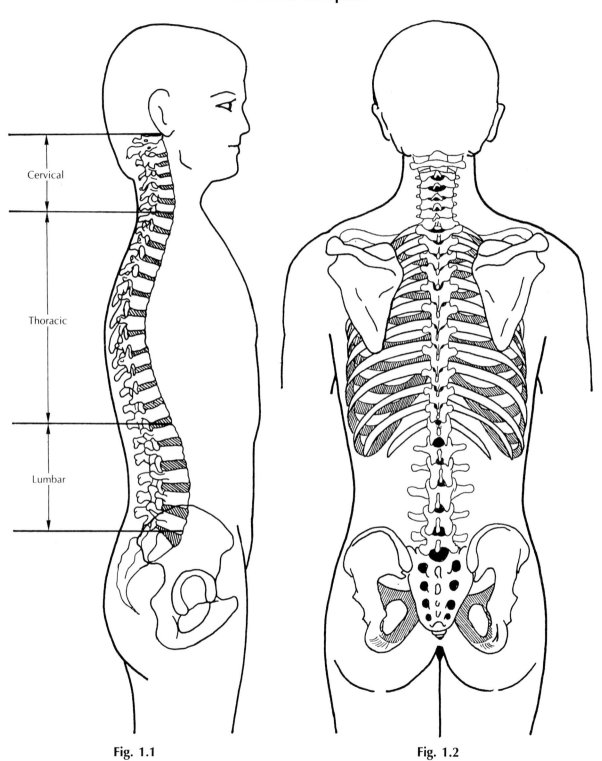

Cervical

Thoracic

Lumbar

Fig. 1.1

Fig. 1.2

Structure of a Motion Segment

The vertebral column consists of a series of motion segments which, when healthy, work in harmony with one another. In order to understand how the whole spine works, it is first necessary to understand the mechanics of the individual motion segment.

A typical motion segment consists of the parts briefly described below (Fig 1.3 is an anatomical illustration and Figs 1.4, 1.6 and 1.7 show a simplified, step-by-step composition).

The intervertebral disc

The anterior part of the motion segment consists of two vertebral bodies and an interposed intervertebral disc (Figs. 1.3 and 1.4), which are the main components in the transmission of loads, including body weight, from one vertebral body to the next. By separating the vertebrae, the disc also allows movement to occur, and the combined movements of all the motion segments in the spine augment those of the limbs.

Each disc has two main components: an outer annulus fibrosus and an inner nucleus pulposus (*see* Fig. 1.8). The annulus fibrosus consists of concentric layers of collagen fibres running in an alternating oblique direction (*see* Fig. 1.9), bound together by a proteoglycan gel. The nucleus pulposus is a semifluid gel containing a higher percentage of proteoglycans than the annulus; these molecules have the property of imbibing fluid – and with it, nutrition—into the disc. In the lumbar region, the nucleus is situated more posteriorly; hence, the annulus in this area of the disc is thinner, especially posterolaterally, where at least 40% of the annular layers are incomplete (Marchand and Ahmed, 1990), constituting a weakness in the disc.

There is always an intrinsic pressure within the discs (intradiscal pressure) even when they are unloaded. This resting pressure rises when the disc is subjected to compression (*see* p. 12) such as from body weight and carrying loads, and also when the disc is flexed (Nachemson, 1965).

The disc is separated from its adjacent vertebral body by two thin end plates (Fig. 1.4) which, during the growth period, are responsible for the longitudinal growth of the vertebral body. The end plates also form a permeable barrier through which water and nutrients can pass from the cancellous bone of the vertebral bodies into the disc. Weakened areas in the end plates left by the involution of blood vessels between 10–15 years of age make the vertebral body vulnerable to *intra*vertebral disc prolapses from the nucleus leaving Schmorl's nodes (*see* pp. 26, 42 and Fig. 2.15).

The neural arch (Fig. 1.5)

Projecting posterolaterally from the upper part of the vertebral body are two stout bones, the pedicles, which together with the laminae—two sheets of bone projecting posteromedially—form the neural arch. The spinous process projects backwards from the junction of the laminae. It is useful to demonstrate to the patient that he can palpate the spinous processes himself as it helps him to appreciate the depth of the different structures in his back. Projecting laterally from the junction of the pedicles and laminae are the transverse processes.

A motion segment

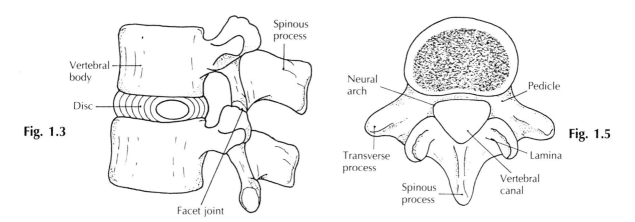

Fig. 1.3

Fig. 1.5

Step-by-step composition

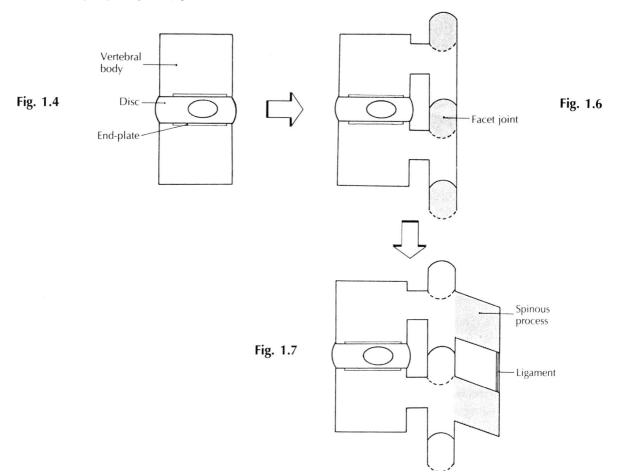

Fig. 1.4

Fig. 1.6

Fig. 1.7

The apophyseal ('facet') joints (Figs. 1.3, 1.6)

Projecting superiorly and inferiorly from the junction of the pedicles and laminae are two articular processes housing articular facets which, with those from adjacent vertebrae, form the apophyseal joints. Being synovial joints, they may incur degenerative changes that are typical of arthrosis. These changes can occur with a relatively normal disc (Lewin, 1964), especially where there is an increased lumbar lordosis and the apophyseal joints bear more weight than normally, but they do not necessarily cause symptoms. More frequently, changes are secondary to degeneration in the disc (*see* p. 32). The capsules of the apophyseal joints are highly innervated, being sensitive to pain, any alteration in direction, speed and degree of movement and changes in atmospheric pressure (Wyke, 1967); in other words, these joints may indeed react to a change in weather conditions. Their structure enables them to guide and restrict movements in order to protect the underlying disc and soft tissues.

The ligaments (Fig. 1.7)

There are numerous ligaments in the spine (*see* 'Further Reading') which subserve the important function of resisting separation of the vertebrae, thereby stabilizing the spine and protecting the underlying structures. Ligaments are highly innervated and can be a source of local and referred pain. Those of hypermobile people (*see* p. 24) are more vulnerable to strain. The transverse and spinous processes give the vertebral column extra leverage, and the ligaments which are attached to the spinous processes are of special significance, especially the supra-spinous and interspinous, which resist separation of the vertebrae during the end phase of spinal flexion. These particular ligaments are relatively weak (Adams *et al.*, 1980) and are, therefore, prone to either rupture, if the limit of flexion is exceeded, or overstretching through sustained flexion postures (*see* p. 22). Research has shown that more than one-fifth of adult lumbar spines have interspinous ligament ruptures (Rissanen, 1960).

The neural tissues

Together with the posterior surfaces of the vertebral bodies, the bony neural arches help to form the vertebral canal (Fig. 1.5) in which lie the spinal cord or, below the level of the L1/2 disc, the cauda equina (the lower lumbar, sacral and coccygeal nerve roots).

Surrounding and protecting the spinal cord and nerve roots are meninges (dura, arachnoid and pia). Normally, these are able to adapt to movements of the vertebral column, but sclerotic or fibrotic lesions may restrict their mobility, giving rise to signs and symptoms of adverse neural tension (*see* 'Further Reading').

Two spinal nerves are given off from the spinal cord segments via ventral and dorsal nerve roots, and are numbered according to the vertebra above them (except in the cervical spine). As the spinal cord is shorter than the vertebral canal in the adult, the length of the nerve roots increases caudally before they reach their intervertebral foramina (Fig. 1.10). Degenerative changes in, for example, the disc or apophyseal joints may decrease the foraminas' dimensions, rendering the nerve roots vulnerable to irritation and compression (Fig. 1.11).

Cross-section through a disc

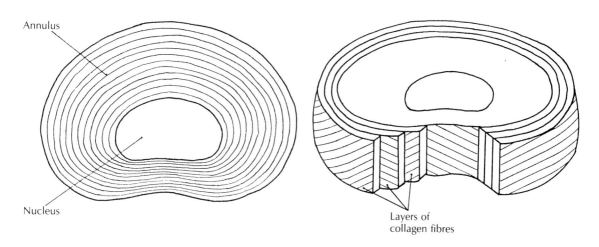

Fig. 1.8

Fig. 1.9

Nerve compression

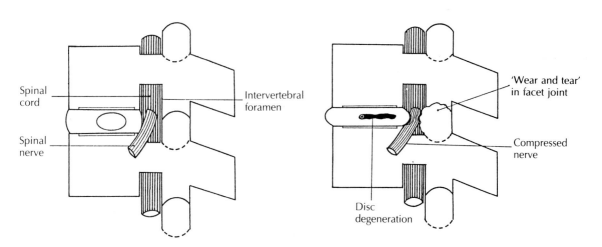

Fig. 1.10   Normal spine.

Fig. 1.11   Degeneration in spine.

The intervertebral foramina are naturally smaller in the lower cervical and low lumbar spine and are, therefore, particularly at risk.

After its exit from the foramen, the spinal nerve supplies a meningeal branch, known as the sinuvertebral nerve (Williams and Warwick, 1986) which re-enters the vertebral canal to supply the dura, blood vessels, periosteum, ligaments and disc. The spinal nerve then divides into ventral and dorsal rami. The larger, ventral rami have connections with the sympathetic nervous system. In the cervical, thoracic and sacral regions, the rami form plexuses, the emerging nerves supplying muscles (*see* Table 1, p. 16 for muscles to be tested for each spinal level), skin (*see* pp. 15, 17 for dermatomes) and bone in the limbs and anterolateral aspects of the trunk. In the thoracic region, the ventral rami are independent of each other. The smaller, dorsal rami supply the muscles and skin on the back of the neck and trunk and apophyseal joints.

The size of the vertebral canal affects the amount of space available for the neural elements within it. Narrowing of the canal, spinal stenosis, (Figs. 1.12, 1.13) may occur, most commonly in the low lumbar spine. It can be congenital, or acquired through encroachment into the canal of osteophytes from the apophyseal joints or vertebral bodies, or because of a bulging or prolapsed disc, or through other degenerative disease processes such as a buckled ligamentum flavum (the ligament connecting adjacent laminae). Symptoms may be felt in the back and legs from compression of the cauda equina, and neurogenic claudication may occur, made worse by walking.

The muscles
(Figs. 1.14, 1.15)

Surrounding the vertebral column is the musculature which produces or controls spinal movements. The small, deep muscles attached to the posterior elements control the intersegmental movements. They provide the stability necessary for the larger, more superficial muscles to produce the grosser spinal movements. The back extensors lie more or less longitudinally and, on contraction, they exert a compressive force on the discs, raising intradiscal pressure in proportion to the strength of their contraction (Fig. 1.15). Many patients will be unaware of the fact that it is not just the muscles behind the trunk that are involved in spinal dysfunction: the abdominal muscles situated anterolaterally play an important role in spinal mechanics. While the back extensors may shorten and tighten in response to spinal dysfunction, there is reciprocal inhibition and weakening of the abdominals.

A degree of muscle spasm is always present with acute back pain and frequently indicates underlying joint dysfunction. However, nervous tension increases the resting level of contraction in muscles, and this is perhaps more evident in the neck muscles, which are more sensitive to anxiety states because they contain a higher proportion of afferent fibres compared with most other striated muscles (Abrahams, 1977). The commonest site for this is at the attachment of the neck muscles to the occiput. Relaxation techniques often have an important part to play in the management of such patients' neck complaints.

Spinal stenosis

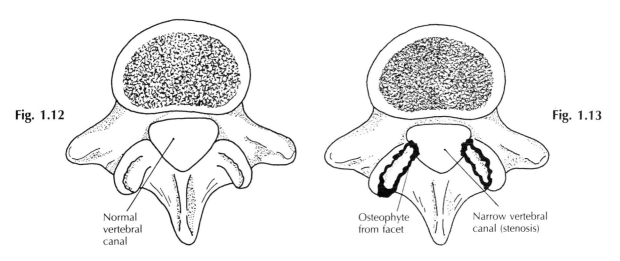

Fig. 1.12

Normal
vertebral
canal

Fig. 1.13

Osteophyte
from facet

Narrow vertebral
canal (stenosis)

Effect of muscle contraction

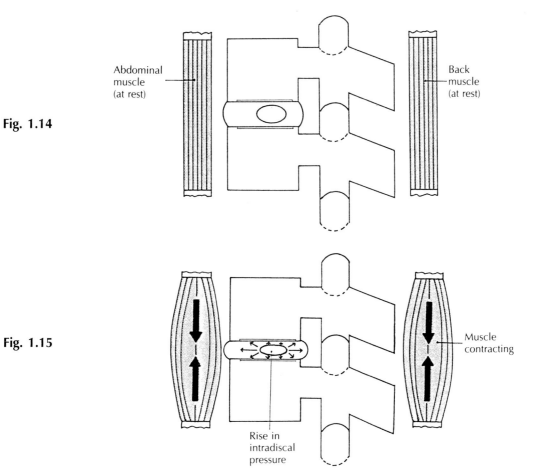

Abdominal
muscle
(at rest)

Back
muscle
(at rest)

Fig. 1.14

Fig. 1.15

Muscle
contracting

Rise in
intradiscal
pressure

Movements of the Spine

Spinal movements occur mainly to augment those of the arms and legs or, in the case of the cervical spine, to position the head to the advantage of the sense organs. Generally, people are less aware of moving their spines than, for example, moving their arms, unless they are reminded of it because of pain.

The basic movements of the lumbar spine are summarized below, but it should be borne in mind that everyday activities such as getting in and out of a car may incur complex combinations of all the spinal movements. It may be necessary to analyse a particular activity that is provoking the patient's pain to discover exactly why it is happening, i.e. the combination of movements involved, compressive factor, length of time required to provoke the symptoms, etc. Hand dominance often has a significant effect on the way people perform activities; extreme right- or left-handedness can lead to problems of both joint and muscle imbalance.

Flexion

Flexion (Figs. 1.16, 1.17) stretches and thins the posterior annular fibres so that the position of the nucleus becomes relatively more posterior. The inferior articular facets of one vertebra glide upwards on the superior articular facets of the one below. Flexion increases both the height of the intervertebral foramina and the length of the posterior border of the vertebral canal. The movement is progressively braked by the supraspinous and interspinous ligaments, the ligamenta flava and the apophyseal joint capsules, but ceases because of the apposition of the superior and inferior articular facets of the apophyseal joints (Twomey and Taylor, 1983). As previously stated, after the limit of flexion is exceeded, the supraspinous and interspinous ligaments are the most vulnerable to sprain (Adams et al., 1980).

What happens during *repetitive* or *sustained flexion* is often more significant than during a single flexion movement. Most activities of modern daily life involve more flexion than extension. It is this tendency which is a hazard to so many backs. Repetitive flexion movements produce creep in the ligaments, increasing the normal range of flexion. Experiments on cadaveric lumbar discs (Adams and Hutton, 1983) have demonstrated that when subjected to repetitive flexion and compression to simulate a vigorous day's activities, some of them showed distortion of the annular lamellae, which became tightly curved and packed together in the posterolateral corners (Fig. 1.18). This could be sufficient in some discs for nuclear or annular material to migrate down these, developing radial fissures (Adams and Hutton, 1985).

Extension

In extension (Figs. 1.19, 1.20), the posterior annular fibres are compressed while the anterior fibres are stretched. The position of the nucleus becomes relatively more centralized. Depending on structural variations, extension is resisted either by bony impact of the inferior facets of the apophyseal joints on the laminae of the vertebra below or by trapping of the interspinous ligament between the spinous processes. The height of the intervertebral foramina is reduced, and the length of the posterior border of the vertebral canal is decreased.

Effect of movements on the spine

Forward bending

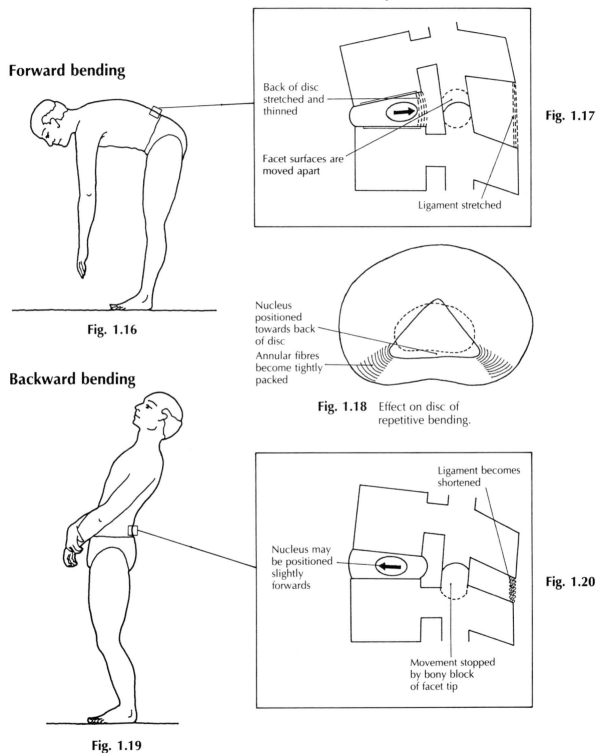

Fig. 1.16

Back of disc stretched and thinned

Facet surfaces are moved apart

Ligament stretched

Fig. 1.17

Nucleus positioned towards back of disc

Annular fibres become tightly packed

Fig. 1.18   Effect on disc of repetitive bending.

Backward bending

Fig. 1.19

Ligament becomes shortened

Nucleus may be positioned slightly forwards

Movement stopped by bony block of facet tip

Fig. 1.20

Rotation

Rotation is normally combined with lateral flexion. The outer annular fibres lying in the direction of the movement are stretched (Fig. 1.21), but rotation is resisted principally by impaction of the inferior articular facet on the opposite side against its subjacent superior articular facet. Only about 3° of rotation to each side can normally occur at each level in the lumbar spine. Beyond this degree, the collagen fibres in the disc undergo microinjury (Hickey and Hukins, 1980). Degenerative changes with thinning of the cartilage lining the apophyseal joints may allow additional rotation (Adams and Hutton, 1981); also, flexion in addition to rotation reduces the locking mechanism of the joints and may allow more movement.

Patients often cite twisting as the movement which injured their backs, but on further questioning, what they often describe is a combination of flexion and lateral flexion (Fig. 1.22).

Lateral flexion

This is a complex movement which is coupled with rotation to the opposite side between L1–4 and to the same side at L5/S1. On the side to which movement occurs, the annulus bulges and the height of the intervertebral foramen is reduced while, on the opposite side, the annular attachments are stretched and the height of the foramen is increased.

Compression on the Spine

When a disc is compressed, the annular fibres and vertebral end plates bulge slightly outwards, and the nucleus deforms radially to dissipate the forces (Figs. 1.23, 1.24). There is a slight loss of disc height, and intradiscal pressure rises in proportion to the amount of compressive force.

Compression occurs in the spine whenever the body is upright, and varies in different postures (*see* p. 31), largely depending on the amount of muscle action used to maintain a particular posture. The spinal muscles are arranged principally in a longitudinal direction so that, when a muscle group contracts, it exerts a compressive force on the spine. Additional loading incurred through lifting or carrying weights increases muscle activity and, therefore, intradiscal pressure depending on the amount of load and distance from the body (*see* p. 108 and Figs. 4.1–4.3).

Prolonged or repetitive loading which may occur during activities such as gardening or during building work leads to increased annular bulging. Fluid is expressed from the discs into the vertebral bodies and surrounding tissues until the discs are in equilibrium with the applied load. Changes in the fluid content of the disc affect its mechanical responses to bending and compression. Degenerated discs show increased bulging, and there is a greater loss of disc height after prolonged loading. This results in an increase in pressure between the facets of the apophyseal joints (Adams and Hutton, 1983) predisposing them to degenerative changes (Fig. 1.25). The dimensions of the intervertebral foramina are also reduced which may jeopardize their contents including the nerve roots.

Unloading the spine, for example by sleeping or resting in crook lying, allows fluid to re-enter the disc and its height to recover.

Effect of movements on the spine

Turning

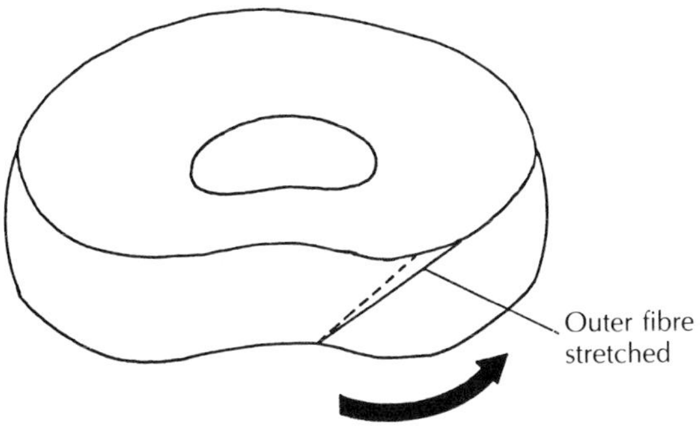

Fig. 1.21

Outer fibre stretched

Bending and turning

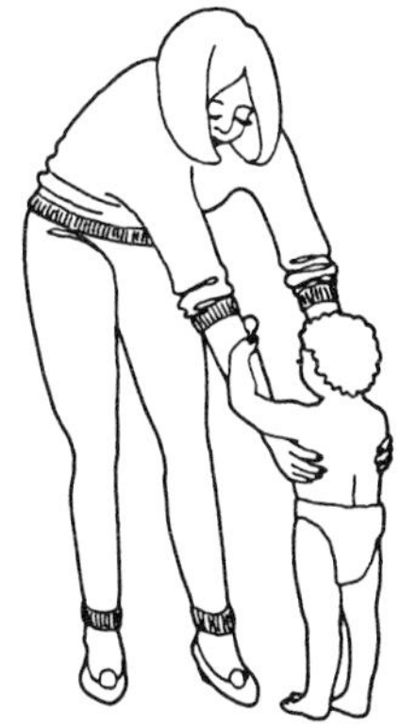

Fig. 1.22

Compression

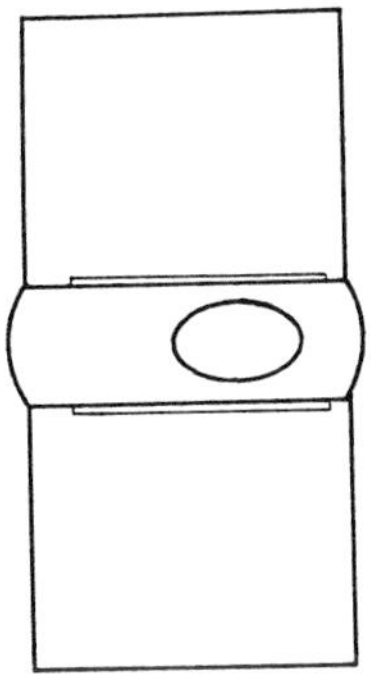

Fig. 1.23 Normal disc at rest.

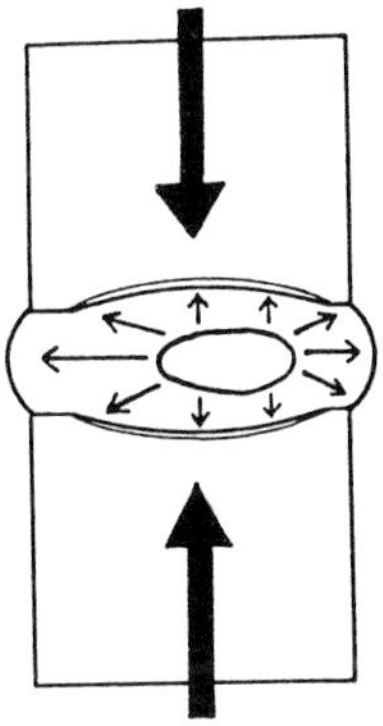

Fig. 1.24 Normal disc under compression.

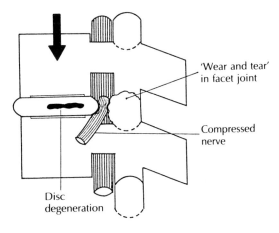

'Wear and tear' in facet joint

Compressed nerve

Disc degeneration

Fig. 1.25 Degenerated spine under compression.

Pain

The spine has an abundant nerve supply and, consequently, pain may arise from most of its musculoskeletal structures, notably the apophyseal joint capsules, ligaments, muscles, cancellous bone, blood vessels, and the anterior aspect of the dura. The disc itself is rather more sparsely innervated, nerve endings having been found in the outer one-third of the annulus (Malinsky, 1959). Whenever nociceptive nerve endings in these structures are irritated, in addition to pain being felt locally, it may also be felt at some distance from them, i.e. 'referred' pain. It is described as a deep, diffuse ache. Usually, the more intense the stimulation of nociceptive nerve endings, the further away from its source the pain appears to spread (Figs. 1.26, 1.27). There is considerable overlap in the areas of referred pain from each segment and inconsistency in the location of referred pain in different individuals, so that the area of referred pain is not diagnostic of a particular level. Adhesions affecting the neuromeningeal structures in one area of the spine can give rise to symptoms at some distance from the original lesion due to their restricted mobility and adverse tension.

Compression of a spinal nerve does not necessarily cause pain (Lindahl, 1966). The pain that may accompany nerve root compression ('radicular' pain) is often described as 'shooting' and linear, and this may be due to a combination of compression and inflammation (Howe, 1979). Radicular pain is generally worse distally, and its distribution is more clearly demarcated within the dermatome of the affected nerve root (Figs. 1.28, 1.29). The pain may also be accompanied by some or all of the following neurological signs:

- *Impaired sensation* and *paraesthesiae* in the area of skin supplied, i.e. the dermatome (Figs. 1.28, 1.29). There are individual variations and overlapping of areas.
- *Weakness* (not usually paralysis unless several spinal nerves are affected) of the muscles supplied by the affected spinal nerve. (Table 1 shows representative muscles to be tested for each segmental level).
- *Reflexes* may be diminished or absent (*see* Table 1). In itself, an absent reflex is not diagnostic of recent spinal nerve root compression; the nerve root may never have recovered from a previous episode of compression.

'Referred' pain

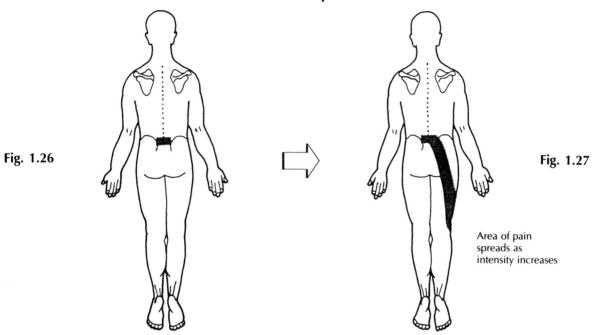

Fig. 1.26

Fig. 1.27

Area of pain
spreads as
intensity increases

Areas of pain from nerve root disorders

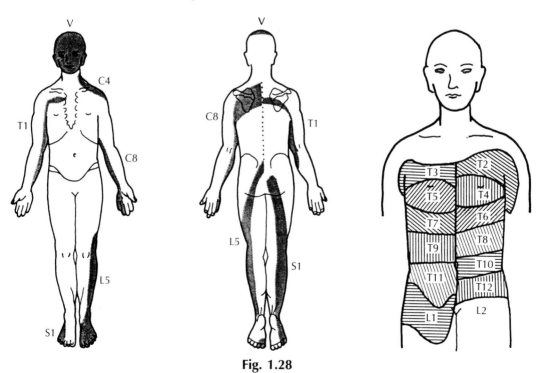

Fig. 1.28

Table 1.1 Nerve Root Supply

Spinal cord segment	Representative muscle(s)	Joint action	Reflex
C1	a.p.r. C1–2 Rect. cap. ant. Longus capitis	Tuck chin in	
C2	p.p.r. C1–2 Rect. cap. post. maj. & minor Obliquus sup.	Push chin up	
C3	a.p.r. C3–4 Scaleni	Press head and neck laterally	
C4	a.p.r. C4 Levator scap. Trapezius	Elevate shoulder girdle	
C5	Deltoid	Abduction of arm	Biceps jerk

C6	Biceps	Elbow flexion	Biceps and
			  brachiora-
			  dialis
			  jerks

C7	Triceps	Elbow extension	Triceps jerk
C8	Thumb extensor Finger flexor	Thumb extension Finger flexion	
T1	Intrinsic hand muscles	Finger adduction and abduction	
L2	Psoas-iliacus	Hip flexion	
L3	Quadriceps	Knee extension	Knee jerk
L4	Tibialis anterior	Foot dorsiflex.	Knee jerk
L5	Extensor hallucis longus	Ext. big toe	
	Extensor digitorum brevis Peronei	Ext. toes Eversion of foot	
S1	Gluteus maximus Hamstrings Calf	Buttock contrac. Knee flex. Toe standing	Ankle jerk
S2	Hamstrings Calf	Knee flexion Toe standing	

Information obtained from the Royal National Orthopaedic Hospital, 1993.

Areas of pain from nerve root disorders

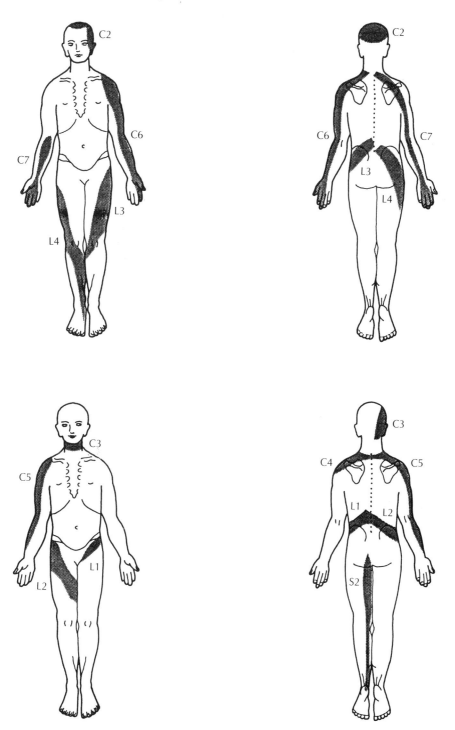

Fig. 1.29

References

Abrahams V. C. (1977). The physiology of neck muscles; their role in head movement and maintenance of posture. *Can. J. Physiol. Pharmacol.*, **55**, 332.

Adams M. A., Hutton W. C., Stott J. R. R. (1980). The resistance to flexion of the lumbar intervertebral joint. *Spine*, **5**, 3, 245.

Adams M. A., Hutton W. C. (1981). The relevance of torsion to the mechanical derangement of the lumbar spine. *Spine*, **6**, 3, 241.

Adams M. A., Hutton W. C. (1983). The effect of fatigue on the lumbar intervertebral disc. *J. Bone Jt. Surg.*, **65-B**, 2, 199.

Adams M. A., Hutton W. C. (1985). Gradual disc prolapse. *Spine*, **10**, 6, 524.

Farfan H. F. (1973). *Mechanical Disorders of the Low Back*. Philadelphia: Lea and Febiger.

Hickey D. S., Hukins D. W. L. (1980). Relation between the structure of the annulus fibrosus and the function and failure of the intervertebral disc. *Spine*, **5**, 2, 106.

Howe J. F. (1979). A neurophysiological basis for the radicular pain of nerve root compression. In *Advances in Pain Research and Therapy*. (Bonica J. J., ed.) New York: Raven Press.

Kapandji I. A. (1974). *The Physiology of the Joints. 3: The Trunk and the Vertebral Column*. Edinburgh: Churchill Livingstone.

Lewin T. (1964). *Osteoarthrosis in Lumbar Synovial Joints*. Gothenburg: Orstadius Bokryckeri Aktiebolag.

Lindahl O. (1966). Hyperalgesia of the lumbar nerve roots in sciatica. *Acta Orthop. Scand.* **37**, 367.

Malinsky J. (1959). The ontogenetic development of nerve terminations in the intervertebral discs of man. *Acta Anat.*, **38**, 96.

Marchand F., Ahmed A. M. (1990). Investigation of the laminate structure of lumbar disc anulus fibrosus. *Spine*, **14**, 2, 166.

Nachemson A. (1965). The effect of forward leaning on lumbar intra-discal pressure. *Acta Orthop. Scand.* **35**, 314.

Rissanen P. M. (1960). The surgical anatomy and pathology of the supraspinous and interspinous ligaments of the lumbar spine with special reference to ligament ruptures. *Acta Orthop. Scand.* (Suppl), 46.

Twomey L. T., Taylor J. R. (1983). Sagittal movements of the human vertebral column: a quantitative study of the role of the posterior vertebral elements. *Arch. Phys. Med. Rehab.*, **64**, 322.

Williams, P. L., Warwick R. (eds.) (1986). *Gray's Anatomy*. Edinburgh: Churchill Livingstone.

Wyke B. D. (1967). The neurology of joints. *Ann. Roy. Coll. Surg. Engl.*, **41**, 25.

Further Reading

Adams M. A., Hutton W. C. (1983). The mechanical function of the lumbar apophyseal joints. *Spine*, **8**, 3, 327.

Butler D. S. (1991). *Mobilisation of the Nervous System*, Edinburgh: Churchill Livingstone.

Dunlop R. B., Adams M. A., Hutton W. C. (1984). Disc space narrowing and the lumbar facet joints. *J. Bone Jt. Surg.*, **66-B**, 5, 705.

Oliver J., Middleditch A. (1991). *Functional Anatomy of the Spine*. Oxford: Butterworth-Heinemann.

2
Syndromes

Therapists whose experience has been mainly in one field, for example treating chronic, stiff backs, or treating people in one occupation, can be misled into believing that one particular structure (say the disc) is responsible for all patients' problems. Spinal syndromes are rarely as clearcut as we would like them to be, but many do have a pattern which is revealed by careful and objective questioning, and examination of the patient. The most common syndromes likely to be seen in practice are presented in this chapter, with various suggestions as to how they can be managed.

Ligamentous Syndromes

Chronic ligamentous strain of the posterior ligaments of the spine

This is the most common back complaint and yet its management is easy for a motivated patient. Unfortunately, not all sufferers come for treatment and advice early enough, and chronic ligamentous strain often progresses until eventually the underlying disc is damaged. The problem usually starts in children, and is caused by sitting in slumped postures in chairs which are either the wrong height (Fig. 2.1), have the seat sloping backwards, or writing at tables which are too low and flat rather than sloping, both at school and at home. Lack of sporting facilities and a reduction in physical activity perpetuates the situation. Poor postural reflexes are learnt and then later carried into occupational situations. Sustained bending postures in standing likewise cause strain.

PATHOLOGY

The cells and collagen fibres in normal ligament tissue are arranged in an undulating pattern that has been described as its 'crimp' (Dale *et al.*, 1972). This allows slight elongation to occur without damage to its fibres. The collagen fibres are oriented in a roughly parallel fashion along the length of the ligament (Frank *et al.*, 1985) and, when the physiologic limits of its crimp are exceeded, as in sustained flexed postures, the fibres begin to fail microscopically. Elongation of the ligament occurs, which may be irreversible, and its mechanical properties are altered. Movement in excess of normal range then occurs in the motion segment, which places greater stress on deeper structures. Ligaments are richly innervated by nociceptive nerve endings (Wyke, 1976) and sustained stretching causes pain, with reflex contraction of the back muscles and a feeling of stiffness. Pain, felt in the early stages at the end of the school or working week, is felt progressively earlier in the offending posture.

BACK CARE EMPHASIS

- Explanation to patient (Fig. 2.1)
- Correction of furniture dimensions (pp. 78–87).
- Adjustments to furniture and cars (pp. 78–81).
- Posture correction in sitting (pp. 88–9) and standing (pp. 100–2).
- Offset flexed position by exercises (Figs. 5.1–5.4, 5.6, 5.7).
- Encourage physical exercise to gain extension: walking, swimming.

Ligament Strain

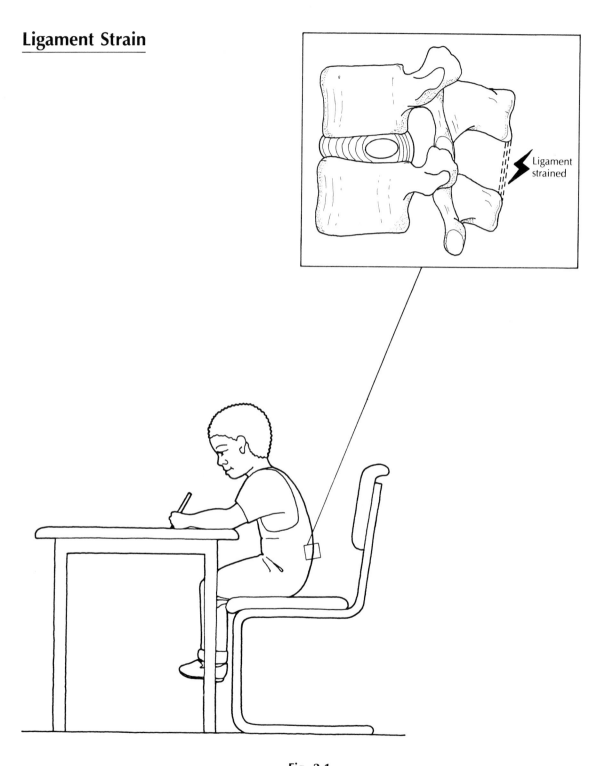

Ligament
strained

Fig. 2.1

Ligament sprains and tears

These can occur in previously normal ligaments, or may be the sequel to the previous syndrome where the ligaments have already been weakened and attenuated. A sprain or tear to the ligaments occurs if a sudden or unexpected stretch is applied (e.g. during sport), especially during the vulnerable recovery phase, or if the ligaments are subjected to sustained pressure or exposed to repeated stress (Hayne, 1987) for example a weekend of gardening or moving house, when an unusual amount of heavy lifting is done.

It is impossible for most people to avoid some degree of spinal flexion when lifting loads from floor level, even when the knees are bent. During the initial lift-off phase, if the weight is over 68.4 kg, the lumbar spine goes into further flexion (Troup, 1979), so if it was already at the end of its normal range of flexion, an additional force of sufficient magnitude, if suddenly applied, would sprain or tear the posterior ligaments. The supraspinous/interspinous ligaments are the first to sprain immediately after the limit of flexion is exceeded (Adams *et al.*, 1980). It has been shown (Rissanen, 1960) that these ligaments have been invariably ruptured or slack in patients presenting for disc surgery. In the early stages it is difficult to distinguish clinically between a ligament sprain and an early low lumbar disc problem.

Repair process

Tearing of ligament fibres leads to haemorrhage, swelling, fibrin formation and the laying down of scar tissue which is mechanically inferior to normal ligament tissue. Proprioceptive feedback from the ligament is also likely to be affected. As ligaments have an abundant supply of nociceptive nerve endings, initially there is localized pain and tenderness with a degree of muscle spasm. During the repair process, pain occurs when the ligament is stretched or compressed. If the new fibres are stretched too soon, this weakens the repair, and elongation of the ligament ensues. Conversely, if movement is not attempted for too long a period, adhesions occur, which consequently stiffen the affected motion segment. Hypermobility at an adjacent segment may be a sequel to this.

BACK CARE EMPHASIS

- Explanation to patient (Fig. 2.2). The lumbar spine when flexed may be likened to a cantilever (Newman, 1968), as seen in some bridges. In a cantilever system (Fig. 2.3), the main horizontal strut is held by a tension support above it and a compression support beneath it. Similarly, the spine acting like the strut is held by the posterior ligaments and muscles, which act as a tension system, and below by the abdominal muscles, which act as a compression system by raising intra-abdominal pressure (Fig. 2.4). The L5/S1 disc acts as the fulcrum of movement.
- Rest is necessary in the early stages: for minor sprains a light corset may be sufficient to provide this; for severe tears bedrest may be needed.
- Correct lying and sitting postures with the lumbar spine in a neutral position to avoid overstretching the ligaments (pp. 67–9, 78–86).
- Advice on lifting (Chapter 4).
- Intermittent stretching once repair is under way to regain length (Figs. 5.16, 5.17, p. 125).

Ligament Sprains and Tears

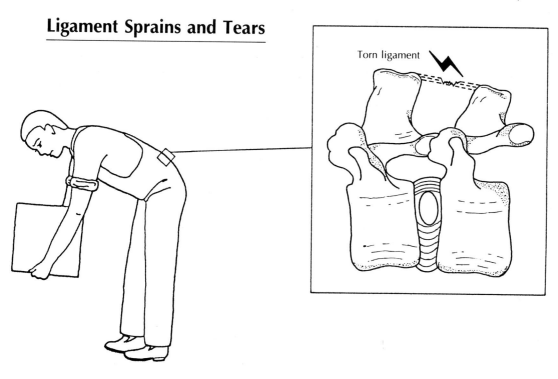

Fig. 2.2   Bending and lifting.

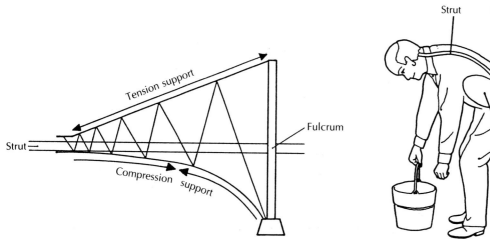

Fig. 2.3   The spine likened to a cantilever system as seen in some bridges (*see* text). (Adapted from P. H. Newman, 1968, The spine, the wood and the trees. *Proc. Roy. Soc. Med.,* **61**, 35.)

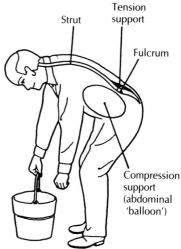

Fig. 2.4

Hypermobility syndrome

Ligaments which are laxer than normal allow an excessive range of movement—hypermobility—at a joint. There is controversy as to whether hypermobility represents the upper end of the normal spectrum of articular movements, or whether it is a distinct, but poorly differentiated, collagen disorder. The majority of people with lax ligaments and loose joints suffer no articular problems. For them, hypermobility is a positive attribute which enables enhanced participation in a variety of physical activities. However, some experience locomotor problems as a direct result of their laxity.

Normal 'tight' ligaments protect joints by acting as a constraint on the range of movements (Adams *et al.*, 1980) and by imposing stability. Lax joints lack such safeguards and are, therefore, more likely to be injured by trauma and overuse. Symptoms arising from lax joints may commence at any age. They occur after, rather than during, unaccustomed exercise (Ansell, 1972) or prolonged stretching. Because detectable clinical abnormalities are often absent, the hypermobility syndrome is underdiagnosed, the patients often being labelled as neurotic. 'Growing pains' in childhood are now being recognized as stemming from hypermobility (Beighton *et al.*, 1983). The ligaments of hypermobile women are more at risk during and shortly after pregnancy because of hormone release which further increases ligamentous laxity (*see* p. 146).

An assessment of a spinal lesion should always include an examination of the ligaments—peripheral as well as spinal. The hypermobile patient often gives a history of being able in his teens to put the palms of his hands flat on the floor during spinal flexion with the knees extended. He may also show excessive movements in the metacarpophalangeal joints and at the elbows and knees. Other members of the patient's family may also be 'double-jointed', as there is a hereditary predisposition, females being more commonly affected than males. Generally, laxity decreases with age. There is a strong clinical impression of a racial variation in joint mobility, Indians and Africans showing more mobility than Europeans (Harris and Joseph, 1949).

PATHOLOGY

Bird *et al.* (1978) drew attention to the way in which joint hyperlaxity may predispose to a traumatic synovitis in the third decade and premature osteoarthrosis in the 4th or 5th. Pyrophosphate is subsequently deposited in the unstable joint. The cervical spine is one of the commonest sites to be affected (Kirk *et al.*, 1967). Protective muscle tone in well-exercised individuals helps to stabilize the joints and, provided they are not traumatized, may well lessen the likelihood of osteoarthrosis. Radiological anomalies, including scoliosis and pars interarticularis defects, with or without spondylolisthesis, are more common amongst patients with widespread joint hypermobility (Grahame *et al.*, 1981).

BACK CARE EMPHASIS

- Explanation to patient (Figs. 2.5–2.7).
- Care during pregnancy and after childbirth (Chapter 7).
- Gentle intermittent stretching of the joints, avoiding overstretching.
- Strengthen abdominals (Figs. 5.8, 5.9, 5.21).
- Encourage toning-up exercises, e.g. swimming.
- Advice on lifting and carrying (Chapter 4).

Hypermobility

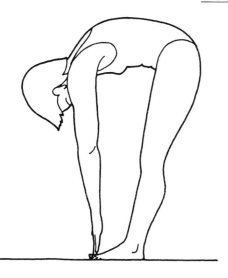

Fig. 2.5 Normal range of forward bending.

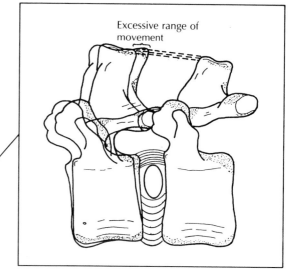

Excessive range of movement

Fig. 2.7

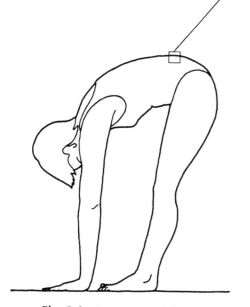

Fig. 2.6 Excessive mobility.

Disc Syndromes

To some patients, the mention of the word 'disc' evokes horrific memories of a friend or relative who had a 'slipped disc' and ended up severely disabled. Therefore, when explaining pathology to the patient, the word should always be used with caution, and never without a full explanation. A reassuring fact is that provided a disc lesion is not allowed to progress beyond Stage 3 (*see* pp. 28–9), bouts of severe, incapacitating pain seldom occur after the age of 55: the changes associated with ageing and degeneration cause the disc to change gradually from having the consistency of the yolk of a 'fried egg' to that of 'crab meat', which is more stable and less likely to herniate.

Causes of disc problems

Hereditary predisposition

There is a strong familial predisposition and the aetiology of degenerative disc disease is related to both genetic and environmental factors (Postacchini *et al.*, 1988). Structural anomalies—such as sacralization (Fig. 2.8), tropism (asymmetrical orientation of apophyseal joints—Fig. 2.9), spondylolysis (defect across the pars interarticularis, without shift of the vertebral body, Fig. 2.10), spondylolisthesis (forward slip of a vertebral body on the one below, Fig. 2.11), a short leg (*see* Figs. 2.74, 2.75)—subject the spine to abnormal stresses which predispose to disc degeneration (Oliver and Middleditch, 1991). Symptoms do not necessarily follow because of the spinal anomaly, but the patient is more at risk because of the prevailing abnormal biomechanics.

Sudden trauma

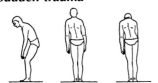

Fig. 2.12 Fig. 2.13 Fig. 2.14

Sudden, severe trauma, such as a too-heavy lift when the spine is in flexion coupled with lateral flexion, can tear the annulus. The patient may feel something 'go' in his back and, classically, is unable to straighten up. Afterwards he may adopt a postural deformity either in flexion (Fig. 2.12), deviated to one side (Fig. 2.13), or a combination of the two (Fig. 2.14). The patient may not have had previous bouts of back pain.

Gradual disc prolapse

More often than not, disc problems are preceded by long periods of ligamentous strain over months or years (*see* 'Ligamentous Syndromes' pp. 20–5). The posterior ligaments, already weakened and attenuated, provide insufficient support, and the stresses eventually fall on the disc. The lower two levels are most commonly affected in the lumbar spine and C5–6 and C6–7 in the cervical spine. What may appear to cause the disc lesion—often a trivial movement such as reaching for the shaving brush—is usually the 'last straw' in a long series of repeated minor traumata.

PATHOLOGY

Changes that occur in the discs do not always follow a clear-cut pattern because structural and mechanical factors are intermingled. Discs can herniate through weakened areas in the end plates into the vertebral body—called *intra*vertebral disc prolapses or Schmorl's nodes (Fig. 2.15), which may be precipitated by heavy axial loading. Radial fissures projecting posteriorly (Fig. 2.16) may create a pathway down which the nuclear and/or annular material may herniate.

Disc Syndromes

Spinal anomalies

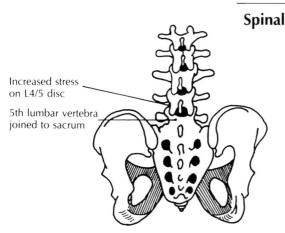

Increased stress
on L4/5 disc

5th lumbar vertebra
joined to sacrum

Fig. 2.8 Sacralization.

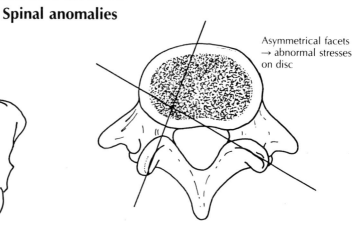

Asymmetrical facets
→ abnormal stresses
on disc

Fig. 2.9 Tropism.

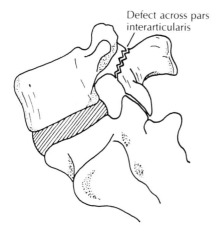

Defect across pars
interarticularis

Fig. 2.10 Spondylolysis.

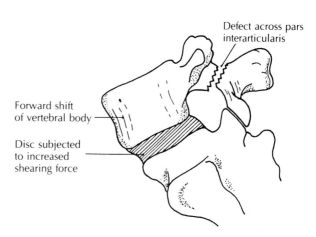

Defect across pars
interarticularis

Forward shift
of vertebral body

Disc subjected
to increased
shearing force

Fig. 2.11 Spondylolisthesis.

Pathological changes in discs

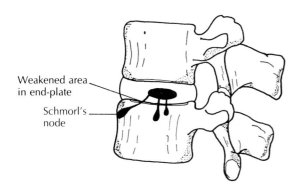

Weakened area
in end-plate

Schmorl's
node

Fig. 2.15

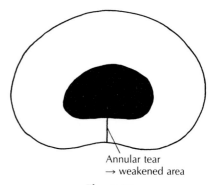

Annular tear
→ weakened area

Fig. 2.16

The gradual posterolateral disc prolapse is the most frequently encountered in clinical practice, and the stages leading up to it are described below.

Stage 1 (Fig. 2.17)

Circumferential tears in the posterolateral area of the disc are usually the first pathological sign. As the disc is poorly innervated except in its outer third (Malinsky, 1959), it is conceivable that some of these tears may be symptomless, or that the symptoms—such as aching or a feeling of 'tiredness' in the back—pass unnoticed. Orientation of the apophyseal joints more in the frontal than in the sagittal plane render them less capable of resisting rotation, and repeated rotatory strains may well cause some of these tears (*see* pp. 12–3).

Stage 2 (Fig. 2.18)

Radial tears emanating from the central nucleus to the periphery of the disc constitute the next stage. Similar tears following distortion of the annular lamellae have been produced experimentally *in vitro* (Adams and Hutton, 1985) by stressing lumbar discs in flexion coupled with lateral flexion and, in some discs, they create a pathway down which nuclear material may track.

Stage 3 (Fig. 2.19)

The nuclear material has tracked down a radial tear to the posterolateral aspect of the disc. The outermost layers of the annulus are still intact. Although this disc may bulge more than a healthy disc on compression, it still retains its hydrostatic properties. Intermittent pressure on a nerve root may occur causing pain, but usually not paraesthesia. Severe bulging may cause a 'sciatic scoliosis' (Fig. 2.13).

Stage 4 (Fig. 2.20)

The nuclear material has herniated through the outer annulus causing irritation and compression of the adjacent nerve root. Severe pain is experienced in a dermatomal distribution (pp. 15,17) and usually, but not always, in the back. Numbness, motor weakness and absent reflexes corresponding to the affected nerve may be immediately apparent or may take several weeks to develop (*see* Table 1, p. 16).

Stage 5 (Fig. 2.21)

Sequestration of the herniated fragment may occur. Occasionally, if the fragment lodges in a non-pain-sensitive area, the pain may miraculously disappear. More commonly, however, it causes adhesions around the nerve, and signs and symptoms of adverse neural tension.

Site of pain

Stages 1–2 (Fig. 2.22)

The patient initially experiences either central or unilateral low back pain or discomfort. Some minor annular tears are undoubtedly symptomless because of the sparsity of nociceptive nerve endings in the disc.

Stage 3 (Fig. 2.23)

With increasing amounts of disc bulging and irritability of the spinal nerve root, the pain is felt more distally. The severity of pathology and the prognosis are worse if the distal pain is greater than that felt proximally. Patients with pain spreading not lower than the knee joint, or with pain that diminishes below the knee joint, can benefit tremendously from following the correct back care advice to prevent the lesion getting worse.

Stages 4–5 (Fig. 2.24)

Referred pain is felt below the knee and possibly into the foot.

Disc Syndromes

Stages leading to disc prolapse

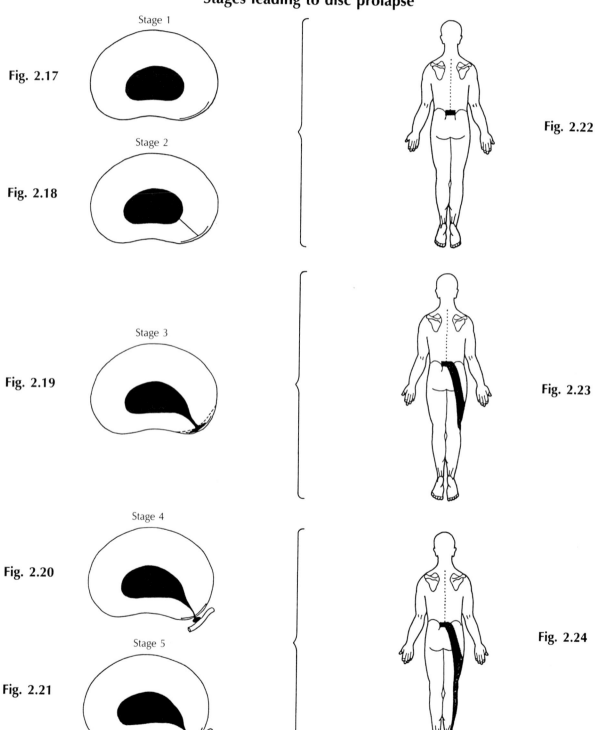

Stage 1

Fig. 2.17

Stage 2

Fig. 2.18

Fig. 2.22

Stage 3

Fig. 2.19

Fig. 2.23

Stage 4

Fig. 2.20

Stage 5

Fig. 2.21

Fig. 2.24

Recovery

Stages 1–3

Initially, the lesion heals by the formation of collagenized scar tissue in the outer annulus only which is *very weak*, and this is why recurrences are common if the patient unduly stresses the disc. The inner annular layers do not heal because they are avascular. Gradual stretching of the scar tissue helps to prevent dysfunction.

Stages 4–5

Surgery may be indicated at this stage. Without it, recovery is very slow and may only be partial. Adhesions, when chronic, can sometimes be successfully stretched.

BACK CARE EMPHASIS

- Explanation to patient:
  Structure of the disc (p. 4 and Figs. 1.8, 1.9);
  Pathology (Figs. 2.16–2.24);
  Disc pressures in different positions (Figs. 2.25, 2.26);
  Dermatomes (Figs. 1.28, 1.29, pp. 15, 17).
- If the lesion is severe, advice on bedrest (pp. 72–5).
- Sitting. At first, sitting may be intolerable as it causes a rise in intradiscal pressure. Symptoms are felt while sitting, or the following morning if the sitting period on the previous day was excessive. Sitting with the lumbar spine flexed further increases intradiscal pressure and, during the acute phase, the patient is usually more comfortable with the lumbar spine in some extension (*see* p. 81) either sitting on a wedge to tilt the pelvis forwards and extend the lumbar spine and/or with a lumbar support. Rising from sitting raises the intradiscal pressure and is painful: arm rests are helpful. The patient should sit only to the point of discomfort, and then should either lie down or walk about.
- Driving—car adaptation (pp. 90–1).
- Exercise—Stages 1–3. It must be remembered that any muscle activity increases intradiscal pressure, and some exercises do so, of course, more than others.
  Acute phase: With severe lesions, if the patient lives alone and has difficulty even turning over into prone, it is inadvisable for him to attempt any specific back exercises. Static quadriceps exercises, foot circling, etc. make the patient feel that he is doing something positive to aid his recovery and will possibly help gently to mobilize the nerves. Teaching the patient diaphragmatic breathing is invaluable in inducing relaxation.
  Subacute phase: When the patient is able to lie prone, an extension regime often helps (*see* Figs. 5.1–4, 5.6, 5.7). Swimming the crawl should be encouraged, or floating/backstroke, as this provides a 'water corset' for the patient and the gentle, symmetrical rotation in extension can be extremely beneficial. As recovery proceeds, flexion, rotation and lateral flexion exercises may be gradually introduced as well as an abdominal strengthening regime (Figs. 5.8, 5.16, 5.17).
- Lifting (*see* also Chapter 4). The patient should not lift in the acute phase, and even later, when taught the correct techniques, he must respect his limitations.
- Danger times. This type of back is often at risk of injury from bending stresses in the *early morning* due to increased fluid content in the disc, especially if combined with high compressive forces (Adams *et al.*, 1987).

Disc Syndromes

Disc pressures

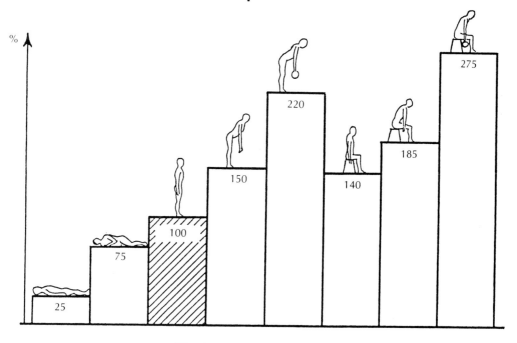

Fig. 2.25 In various positions.

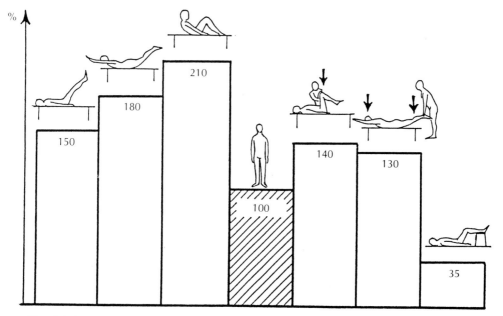

Fig. 2.26 In various muscle strengthening exercises. (Both Figs 2.25 and 2.26 show the relative change in pressure (or load) in the 3rd lumbar disc. From A. Nachemson, 1976. The lumbar spine: an orthopaedic challenge. *Spine*, **1**, 59–71, with permission of author and publisher, Harper and Row.)

Facet Syndrome

Symptoms arising from the apophyseal (facet) joints are more common at the lower two lumbar levels in people over the age of 45, but may be present in the 20s or 30s, when the upper lumbar levels are more frequently affected. These joints, being synovial, are subject to arthrotic changes similar to those occurring in peripheral synovial joints. This is more likely:

if the joints are traumatized—the capsular ligaments are most likely to be damaged in flexion combined with lateral flexion (Adams and Hutton 1983);
in patients with particular postures such as an excessive lordosis (*see* pp. 40–1);
in occupations that involve loading the spinal joints in extension;
in patients with a familial predisposition;
as a sequel to hypermobility (*see* pp. 24–5).

Changes in the apophyseal joints are more commonly secondary to degenerative changes in the disc, especially if the disc space is narrow causing subluxation of the facets (Figs. 2.27, 2.28). Patients who undergo disc excision or chemonucleolysis which results in disc space narrowing face the consequences of a marked increase in pressure across the apophyseal joints (Dunlop *et al.*, 1984).

PATHOLOGY

An acute injury to an apophyseal joint causes synovial effusion, histamine release, stretching or tearing of the capsule and ligaments, and bleeding. Together with protective muscle spasm, this causes a reduction in movement in the joint which may persist if the injury has been severe. Repetitive stresses may lead to a chronic synovial reaction with fraying and fragmentation of the articular cartilage, forming loose bodies. Later the capsule becomes lax, allowing subluxation of the joint surfaces to occur. Marginal osteophytes form which may project into the spinal canal or intervertebral foramina (Fig. 2.29). Finally, the capsule thickens and intra-articular adhesions form across the articular surfaces, further limiting movements.

Areas of pain

Low back pain is initially experienced over the affected joint/s, spreading, if more severe, into the groin, buttock or thigh (Figs. 2.30, 2.31), but not usually below the knee. If, however, there is gross distension and thickening of the capsule, the spinal nerve emerging through the intervertebral foramen may be irritated and/or compressed, giving rise to symptoms more distally.

Typically, symptoms are increased when the apophyseal joints are compressed such as in extension or lateral flexion to the ipsilateral side.

BACK CARE EMPHASIS

- Explanation to patient (Figs 2.27–2.32). It is advisable to use the term 'wear and tear' to the patient, which is accurate and sounds less sinister than 'arthritis'; patients often consider the latter to be a progressive and crippling disease.
- Posture correction. Combined with an excessive lordosis, the patient may also have increased thoracic and cervical curves, internally rotated hips and flat feet (Fig. 2.32). Other joints, e.g. knees, may also have degenerative changes which need to be taken into consideration.

   First the patient needs to be taught to flatten the low back (*see* pelvic tilting regime, Figs. 5.8–5.11) and then to correct his whole spinal posture (*see* pp. 100–2).

Facet Syndrome

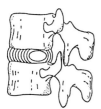

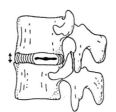

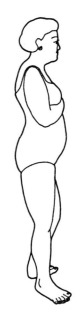

Fig. 2.27   Normal disc space.

Fig. 2.28   Narrow disc space causing subluxation of facets.

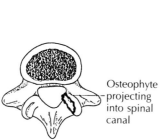

Osteophyte projecting into spinal canal

Fig. 2.29

Fig. 2.32   Facet syndrome: increased spinal curves.

Areas of referred pain from facet joints

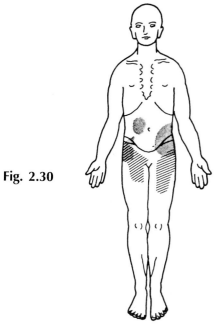

Fig. 2.30

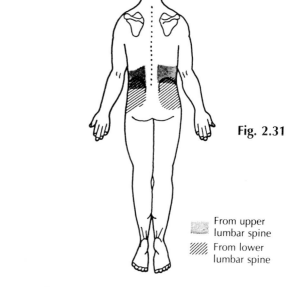

Fig. 2.31

From upper lumbar spine
From lower lumbar spine

(Both Figs 2.30 and 2.31 adapted from I. W. McCall, W. M. Park and J. P. O'Brien, 1979. Induced pain referral from posterior lumbar elements in normal subjects. *Spine,* **4**, 5, 441.)

Whenever the arms are raised above shoulder height, the patient should learn to prevent latissimus dorsi pulling the lumbar spine into extension, by tilting his pelvis backwards, e.g. when opening windows or hanging out clothes (Fig. 2.33).

- Advice on standing. In prolonged standing, the lumbar spine falls into more extension and the apophyseal joints then take more weight. The patient should try one of the following:

  1. Stand with one leg forward and that knee slightly bent, and gently rock from one foot to the other (Fig. 2.34).
  2. Tilt the pelvis backwards with the knees slightly bent (Fig. 2.35).
  3. Rest the lumbar spine against a wall with the feet forward (Fig. 2.36).
  4. Put one foot on a low stool (Fig. 2.37).

- Advice on sitting. These patients usually prefer sitting rather than standing, with the lumbar spine in a neutral or slightly flexed position, because this shifts the weight off the apophyseal joints onto the discs. Sitting in extension (e.g. on a kneeling stool — Fig. 2.38) is usually *not* helpful for these patients, and the knees may also be arthrotic. Often the patient prefers sitting with the hips level with the knees or lower, e.g. with the feet on a footstool (Fig. 2.39).

  If the arthrosis is secondary to disc degeneration, sitting for long periods is uncomfortable, and the patient may obtain relief by alternately shuffling the buttocks backwards and forwards, e.g. when in a car.

- Rising from sitting. After prolonged sitting, rising from a chair may be painful, because it normally involves arching the low back. Sitting *too* low makes this even more difficult. It is useful for the patient to practise the correct method slowly (Figs. 2.40–2.42).

- Comfortable resting and sleeping positions. These place the lumbar spine in a neutral or slightly flexed position (Figs. 2.43, 2.44). Sleeping prone places the lumbar spine's apophyseal joints in sustained extension, and the cervical joints on the side to which the head is rotated in compression. It is, therefore, best avoided.

  A firm rather than a very hard bed is usually more comfortable for these patients (pp. 62–4).

- Footwear. This often merits consideration. Generally, too high or too low heels may aggravate the condition. Orthoses often need to be prescribed to correct faulty foot biomechanics.

- Exercises. It is often revealing to check which exercises the patient is already doing: is he following a particular video or tape which involves a lot of backward bending? Performing exercises indiscriminately without testing the effect of each is often harmful. Abdominal strengthening and flexion exercises are usually the most helpful (Figs. 5.8–5.11, 5.16, 5.21), avoiding the bilateral straight-leg-raising exercise from supine, which initially lordoses the lumbar spine. If the facet problem is secondary to disc degeneration, *inner range flexion* may exacerbate the latter. Swimming—the crawl rather than breaststroke is preferable as it avoids jarring the low back into hyperextension.

- Diet. A protruberant abdomen can increase the lumbar lordosis, causing excessive loading through the apophyseal joints. Crash slimming diets should be avoided; a serious, slow, steady weight loss is better.

Facet Syndrome
Pain-relieving standing postures

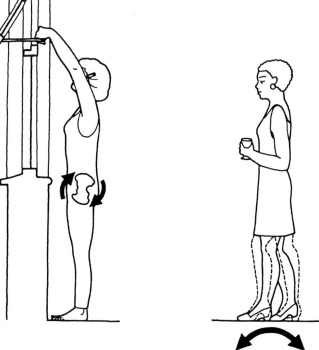

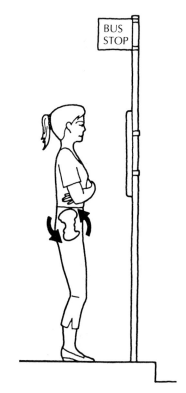

Fig. 2.33 Tilt pelvis backwards.

Fig. 2.34 Rock from one foot to the other.

Fig. 2.35 Tilt pelvis backwards.

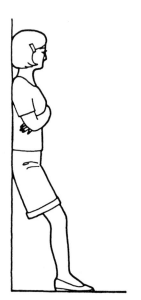

Fig. 2.36 Rest low back against wall.

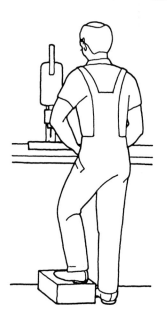

Fig. 2.37 A footstool eases the strain.

Facet Syndrome

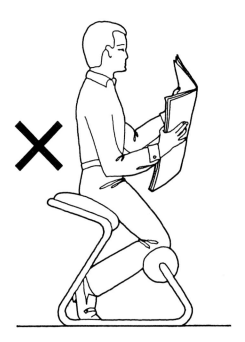

Fig. 2.38   Unsuitable sitting position for this particular syndrome.

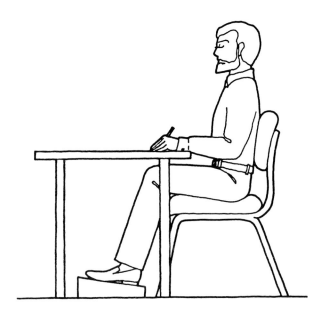

Fig. 2.39   More comfortable position.

Facet Syndrome

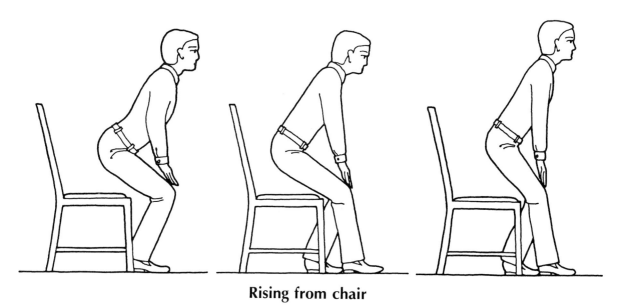

Rising from chair

Fig. 2.40 Avoid arching back.

Fig. 2.41 Bend from hips, keeping tummy tucked in.

Fig. 2.42 Keep low back flat.

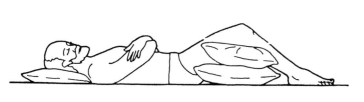

Fig. 2.43

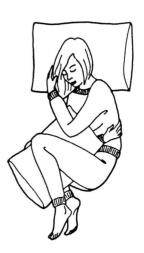

Fig. 2.44

Comfortable resting positions

Sacroiliac Syndrome

Pain in the region of the sacroiliac joint, or even tenderness on palpation, does not necessarily implicate the joint as the source of the pain, because it is the most common site for pain referral from the lumbar spine. The latter, therefore, should first be thoroughly examined before assuming that a lesion is intrinsic to the sacroiliac joint.

Mechanical lesions affecting the sacroiliac joint are ligamentous sprains and/or overriding of the joint. The integrity of the joint principally depends on the strong ligaments which bind it together and the irregularities of the joint's surfaces, the many grooves and depressions of which fit into one another to some extent, increasing its stability. No muscles act as prime movers to the joint, but tension in those muscles passing over it or which attach the pelvis to the trunk or femora, e.g. the abdominal muscles, indirectly impose movement or stresses on the joint.

Women's joints are more susceptible to damage for several reasons. On the whole, their joints have more shallow convolutions, which allow more movement to take place. Also, their ligaments are rendered laxer in pregnancy due to the effect of the hormone relaxin, particularly during the last three months. Return to normal starts soon after delivery, but is not complete until 3–5 months (Abramson *et al.*, 1934). Laxity is more marked in the second pregnancy than the first (*see* also Chapter 7). Ligament sprains associated with pregnancy are the most common cause of sacroiliac joint dysfunction.

In individuals who have a marked forward tilt of the sacrum and an excessive lordosis (Fig. 2.32), the strain on the sacroiliac joints is increased, particularly in the presence of ligamentous laxity (*see* Hypermobility Syndrome, p. 24). The joints can also be sprained by a fall on the side or on the buttocks, the anterior sacroiliac ligament being particularly weak and easily damaged. Torsion of the spine and sacrum with a relatively fixed pelvis can also strain the ligaments, as in the golfer's swing (Fig. 2.45). The presence of a short leg is sometimes an aggravating factor by causing compensatory torsion of the pelvis.

Where overriding of the joint has occurred, it may first need mobilizing or manipulating to 'unhitch' it. The following advice is aimed at preventing recurrent sprains.

BACK CARE EMPHASIS

This should be directed at stabilizing the joints.

- Explanation to patient (Fig. 2.45).
- Advice on avoiding torsional strains such as stepping up onto a chair. (Fig. 2.46). When turning over in bed, the patient should keep the knees together and crooked.
- Use of a heel raise for a short leg (*see* p. 50).
- Use of sacroiliac binder and support during pregnancy (Figs. 7.27, 7.28, p. 157).
- Advice on posture (*see* pp. 100–2), especially backward pelvic tilting to reduce the strain on the sacroiliac joints. Asymmetrical standing (Fig. 2.47) should be avoided.
- See Chapter 7 on care during pregnancy and postnatally.

Sacroiliac Syndrome

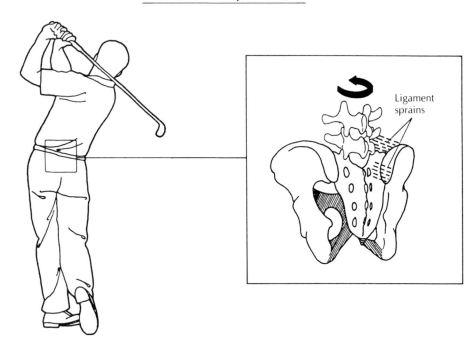

Fig. 2.45

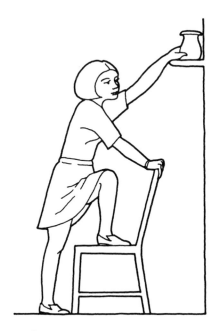

Fig. 2.46 Avoid torsional strain such as this.

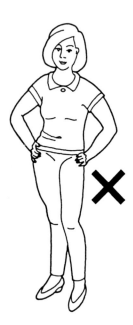

Fig. 2.47 Avoid asymmetrical standing.

Syndromes Related to Structural Faults

Structural faults which cause deviations from the normal curvatures of the spine make it more vulnerable to mechanical stresses. Although not necessarily in themselves the sole cause of pain, they alter the optimum weight distribution through the motion segments and are, therefore, predisposing factors. Normally, weight is transmitted predominantly through the interbody joints, the apophyseal joints playing a relatively minor role in this respect (about 16%, Dunlop *et al.*, 1984). In some conditions, such as increased lordosis or scoliosis, the apophyseal joints may be subjected to greater loading than they are constructed to bear.

Stresses are reduced if the curves are mobile. Pain is not necessarily experienced in the region of the structural fault, but may be at a distance from it due to compensatory mechanisms, e.g. a stiff, kyphotic thoracic spine causing stress in the lumbar spine.

Lordosis

The angle of pelvic tilt is said to be normal in the standing position when the anterior superior iliac spines and the symphysis pubis all lie in the same vertical plane. This gives an angle between the superior surface of the sacrum and the horizontal in the region of 55° (Figs. 2.48, 2.49). An increase in this angle gives rise to an accentuation of the normal lumbar lordosis (Figs. 2.50, 2.51). Lax abdominal muscles and a protruberant abdomen are predisposing factors. Sometimes the increased lordosis is compensatory, balancing a fixed flexion deformity in the hip.

In the standing position, excessive weight then passes through the posterior elements (especially at the lower two lumbar levels), that is, the spinous processes, apophyseal joints, pars interarticularis (Fig. 2.52) and the sacroiliac joints are under increased stress.

Characteristically, backache occurs during activities involving extension of the lumbar spine, such as prolonged standing (which tends to accentuate the lordosis), walking and prone lying. Flexion usually relieves symptoms, so the patient often prefers to sit down or lie in the fetal position.

Sometimes the picture may be complicated by a concomitant disc problem. An accentuated lordosis increases the shearing strain on the lower lumbar discs in the standing position, and degeneration of the posterior annular fibres by 'pressure atrophy' (Lindblom, 1957) may occur as a consequence of this posture.

Area of pain

The pain is usually symmetrical in the low lumbar region, spreading into the sacroiliac region.

BACK CARE EMPHASIS

- Explanation to patient (Figs. 2.48–2.52).
- Correction of forward pelvic tilt (Figs. 5.8–5.11, p. 123).
- Exercises to stretch the lumbar extensors (Fig. 5.16, p. 125) and strengthen the abdominals (Fig. 5.21, p. 128) are often helpful.
- Standing positions to relieve stress (Figs. 3.82, 3.84, 3.88, 3.90, pp. 101, 103, 105). The wearing of high heels sometimes aggravates the condition.
- Comfortable resting and sleeping positions (Figs. 3.10–3.12, 3.15, pp. 68–9).
- Sitting (*see also* pp. 76–89). The patient may be more comfortable with the feet on a footrest, and support low in the back (Fig. 2.53).
- Advice on diet if necessary.

Lordosis

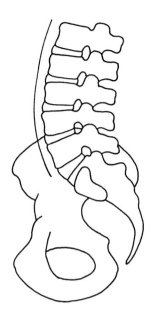

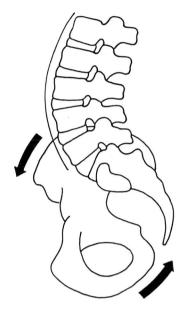

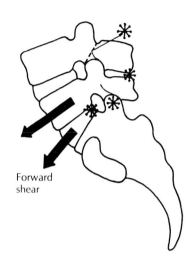

Forward
shear

Fig. 2.48 Normal lordosis.

Fig. 2.50 Increased lordosis.
Pelvis is tilted forwards.

Fig. 2.52 Stress points.

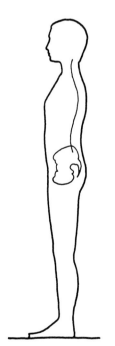

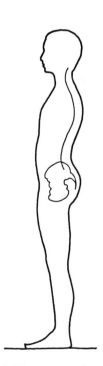

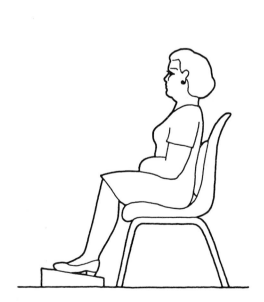

Fig. 2.49 Normal curves. **Fig. 2.51** Increased curves.

Fig. 2.53

Kyphosis

Kyphosis is defined as an abnormal increase in the posterior concavity of the spine. The deformity may take the form of a long rounded curve with its apex at T7–9 (Fig. 2.54), a thoracolumbar kyphosis with its apex at T11–12 or a localized sharp posterior angulation.

Before assuming that a kyphosis is simply due to weak muscles and poor posture, other causes must be considered, so that realistic aims can be set as to how much correction of the curvature is possible. Causes of kyphosis include wedge compression of a vertebral body (which gives the angular type of kyphosis), ankylosing spondylitis, osteochondrosis of the spine, and senile osteoporosis. The latter two are described below.

Osteochondrosis of the spine

This is the term now used for a growth disorder first described by Scheuermann in 1921. It is essentially a degenerative rather than an inflammatory process. There is an alteration in the matrix of the vertebral end plates and the growth plate cartilage due to a change in the collagen: proteoglycan ratio, usually with an increase in the proteoglycans. Ossification of the vertebral body is disturbed, affecting its longitudinal growth, and the cartilage of the end plates is weakened. The normal nutrition of the discs is impaired, and blood vessels grow into the nucleus pulposus, leading to fibrosis and loss of mobility (Stoddard, 1983).

Radiographically, the disease is characterized by the presence of Schmorl's nodes secondary to penetration of nuclear material into the spongiosa of the vertebral bodies (Fig. 2.55), increased anterior wedging of the vertebral bodies (Fig. 2.56), usually (but not always) causing a kyphosis, irregular appearance of the vertebral end plates and, in the later stages, irregular and narrow disc spaces.

The active stage of the disorder starts in the early teens, predominantly near the anterior margins of the vertebrae. Under pressure, the poor quality cartilage tends to collapse, usually resulting in a kyphosis, and the teenager may find it increasingly difficult to maintain a good posture. Although less severe causes may be symptom-free, some teenagers experience intermittent backache, aggravated by contact sports and prolonged flexed postures. The backache is often felt the day following the offending activity. Symptoms usually subside when growth ceases and the affected area is left relatively rigid. Depending on its extent, stiffness in one area of the spine tends to cause hypermobility in adjacent areas, and a compensatory lordosis may develop in the lumbar spine, causing symptoms later in life due to increased mechanical stresses.

BACK CARE EMPHASIS

- Explanation to teenager and parents (Figs. 2.54–2.56), stressing the dangers of excessive weight lifting during the active phase.
- Advice on which sporting activities the teenager should pursue, encouraging swimming, but avoiding sports which jar the spine, such as rugby during the active phase of the disorder.
- Correct sitting posture (*see* p. 88 and Figs. 3.52–3.58).
- Daily gentle stretching over a roll (Fig. 2.57) in lying and over a chair in sitting (Fig. 2.58). Unwanted hyperextension of the lumbar spine is prevented by flexing one hip and knee.

Osteochondrosis (Scheuermann's)

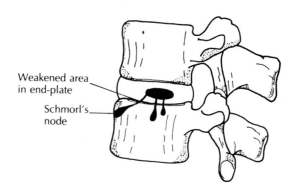

Weakened area
in end-plate

Schmorl's
node

Fig. 2.55 Schmorl's nodes.

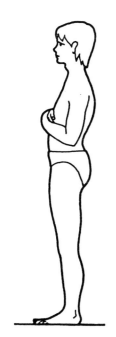

Fig. 2.54 Increased
thoracic curve.

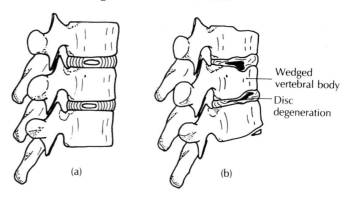

Wedged
vertebral body

Disc
degeneration

(a)   (b)

Fig. 2.56 (a) A normal spine. (b) Scheuermann's.

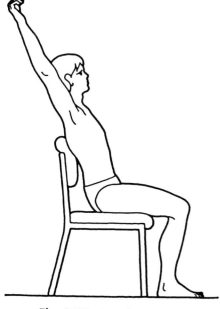

Fig. 2.58 Stretching over
back of chair.

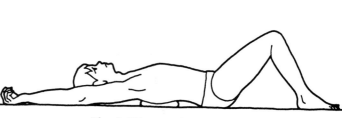

Fig. 2.57 Stretching over a roll.

- An exercise regime to maintain as much movement as is realistically possible in the affected area, bearing in mind the pathological process, and without putting undue strain on adjacent areas of the spine. Fast walking, swinging the arms, is helpful.
- For symptoms arising from a lordotic lumbar spine, *see* pp. 40–1.

Osteoporosis

This is a disease in which bone is lost from the skeleton at a pathological rate. The whole skeleton is affected, but changes in the vertebral bodies are more obvious than elsewhere.

Peak bone mass (Fig. 2.59) is attained at the end of the growth period, and this governs skeletal integrity for the rest of life (Dixon, 1986). With ageing, a degree of bone loss occurs, women being more commonly affected than men, especially a decade or more after the menopause. In women aged 45–55, the rate of bone loss is accelerated, but between one-fifth to one-quarter of them have a catastrophic loss—up to 8%—which renders the vertebrae vulnerable to compression fractures from only trivial trauma. Atrophy of the oblique and horizontal trabeculae of the cancellous bone occurs, and the vertebral bodies tend to collapse anteriorly, which is an area of mechanical weakness. They become wedge-shaped and this can happen even without fracture. A rounded kyphosis with loss of stature results (Fig. 2.60).

The cause of osteoporosis is often complex, but the most important factor is often an endocrine deficiency. Women who have had their ovaries removed are at greater risk. By the time osteoporosis shows up on X-ray, at least one-third to one-half of bone density is reduced.

Although the condition may be symptomless, recurrent episodes of generalized backache are common, often in the low thoracic area and sometimes with girdle pain. The onset may be insidious, unless a compression fracture has occurred, in which case it is sudden and the pain is sharper. Healing may take up to 3 months, although pain usually abates in 3–4 weeks. The kyphosis causes chronic ligamentous strain and muscular fatigue. Those postures which increase compression of the spine—sitting (especially without armrests), standing or walking—often aggravate the pain, whereas lying gives some relief.

There is some evidence to suggest that a suitable exercise programme may improve bone density (Krolner *et al.*, 1983).

BACK CARE EMPHASIS

- Explanation to patient (Figs. 2.59, 2.60). Usually the patient will recognize this condition as 'brittle bones'.
- Encourage rest if appropriate, but if rest in bed is necessary when a fracture has occurred, the period should be kept as short as possible. A pain-relieving position is often crook-lying with a foam roll under the affected area (Fig. 2.61).
- Advice on taking suitable exercise when the acute pain has subsided, because mechanical stresses stimulate bone formation. Moderate and regular exercise is best, including walking, swinging the arms to maintain extension and muscle tone.

Osteoporosis

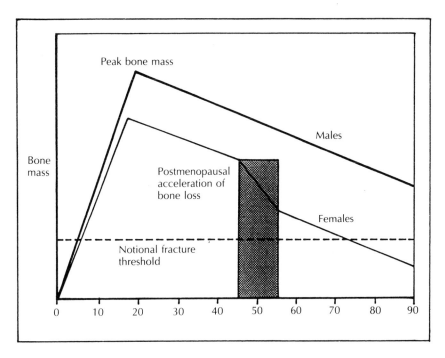

Fig. 2.59   Age-related bone loss from peak bone mass.
(From A. St. J. Dixon, 1986. Osteoporosis – an unheeded epidemic. *Practitioner,* **230**, 363.)

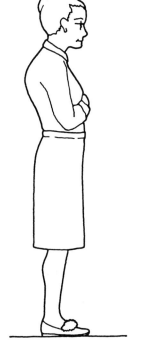

Fig. 2.60   Osteoporotic spine.

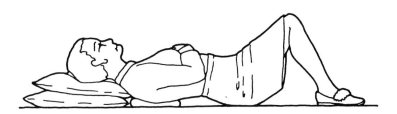

Fig. 2.61   Pain-relieving position.

Scoliosis

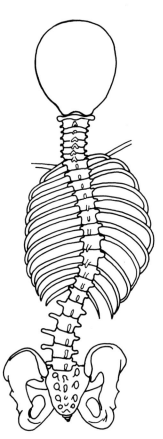

Fig. 2.62

Scoliosis is a lateral curvature of the spine (Figs. 2.62–64) which can either be structural or non-structural. Lateral curves occur more frequently in girls than boys, and there is often a genetic or familial background, but the majority of cases are idiopathic. Quite often a physiotherapist may be the first to detect a curvature, and it is imperative not to alarm the child or parents, who may well remember a relative with an unattractive hump and automatically assume that the child will acquire one.

In *non-structural scoliosis*, there is no fixed rotation of the vertebrae. The curvature may be 'postural', which corrects itself in the lying position, compensatory, e.g. due to leg length inequality, or so-called 'sciatic' (*see* Fig. 3.73, p. 97).

In *structural scoliosis*, there is a fixed rotation of the vertebral bodies towards the convexity, the spinous processes pointing towards the concavity. Compensatory curves occur above and below the structural curve and in an opposite direction to keep the head vertically above the pelvis. The ribs on the convexity are carried backwards with the vertebral body rotation, causing a gibbus (hump), whereas the ribs on the concavity are crowded together forming a costal depression (rib valley), and are carried forwards, so that there may be an anterior protrusion of the chest wall on this side (Figs. 2.63, 2.64). The shoulder girdle is drawn posteriorly above the rib valley, below which is a lumbar hump. On the side of the thoracic hump, the shoulder girdle is drawn anteriorly, and there is a concavity in the lumbar region.

A state of muscle and soft tissue imbalance is present, with short, contracted muscles in the concavities and elongated, overstretched muscles over the convexities (Figs. 2.65–66).

Clinically, identification between the two types of scoliosis is more evident on flexion. With a postural scoliosis any lateral curvature that was present when standing will straighten on flexion, and there will be no persisting rotation. In the structural type, the curve will persist, and dorsal elevations and depressions are apparent (Fig. 2.67).

Unequal leg lengths do not cause a structural scoliosis, but they produce a curve of the spine convex towards the short leg side. When a child has a slight shortening of the leg, which may not even be obvious, on flexion of the trunk an apparent rotation of the lumbar spine will be present. If the pelvis is levelled by placing blocks under the short leg, the apparent rotation disappears.

Progression of the curvatures in scoliosis depends to a large extent on age of onset and magnitude of the angle of curvature. During the adolescent growing period, progression is at a faster rate. Children with structural curves should be referred to an orthopaedic surgeon who will objectively monitor the angle of curvature (Cobb angle—Fig. 2.68) by means of X-rays. In severe cases, surgery may be indicated.

Problems associated with scoliosis are:

- Psychological ones because of the deformity;
- Reduced pulmonary function;
- Pain, especially with increasing age.

Scoliosis

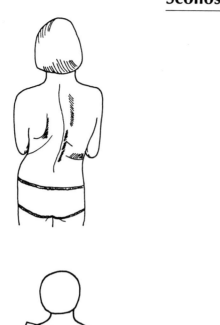

Fig. 2.63

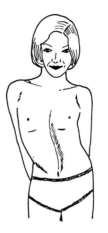

Fig. 2.64

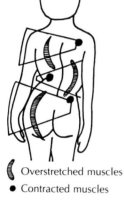

Fig. 2.65

(Overstretched muscles
● Contracted muscles

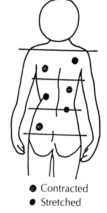

Fig. 2.66

◐ Contracted
● Stretched

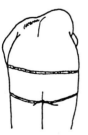

Fig. 2.67 Structural scoliosis:
dorsal elevation evident
on forward bending.

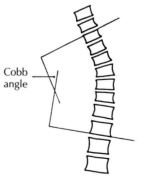

Cobb angle

Fig. 2.68

Both Figs. 2.65 and 2.66 show correction of scoliotic body statics. (From C. Lehnert-Schroth, 1991).

The role of an exercise programme for scoliosis has been controversial. Exercises have in the past been carried out mainly in one plane, and the results of these were often disappointing. However, a three-dimensional approach developed by Katharina Schroth, which is based on sensorimotor and kinaesthetic principles has attracted considerable interest (*see* 'Further Reading'). Each exercise has four components:

1. *Correct starting position*

   The exercises are begun in an asymmetric position designed to maximize correction of the scoliotic posture. Small, firm pads may be used which are strategically placed to stimulate the weak, overstretched muscles (Fig. 2.69). The patient never lies on the side of the thoracic hump as this *increases* the deformity.

2. *Upward elongation*

   For educational purposes, Katharina Schroth divided the trunk into three blocks, each representing the shoulder girdle, rib cage and pelvic girdle. In a normal trunk, the blocks would be above one another (Fig. 2.70), but in a scoliotic spine they are shifted laterally, away from the vertical axis, the shoulder and pelvic girdles in one direction and the rib cage in the opposite direction in both sagittal and frontal planes (Fig. 2.71). The greater the shift from the vertical axis, the more they rotate in the transverse plane (Fig. 2.72). The trunk in effect becomes shorter. Therefore, before performing any of the exercises, active elongation of the trunk is performed in a 'wriggling' motion.

3. *Rotational breathing*

   Rotational breathing plays a vital part in any exercise the patient performs. Through their articulations with the vertebral column, the ribs can reduce torsion in the spine (called derotation). By means of tactile stimulation, initially by the physiotherapist, air is directed to the concave areas of the thorax. Short, explicit verbal commands are used. Breathing bands with which the patient can practise are useful (Fig. 2.73). As well as effecting a reduction in the deformity, greater rib mobility leads to an increase in the patient's vital capacity.

4. *Stabilizing muscle action*

   The patient breathes out as slowly as he can against resistance, using a fff, sss or shshsh sound, at the same time maintaining width over the concave areas by corrective contraction of the rib hump in a forwards and inwards direction.

   Simple equipment such as chairs and tables are used so that the patient, following an intensive treatment programme, can practise at home.

   Corrective exercises with rotational breathing are repeated many times. They facilitate new movement patterns; by consciously repeating derotative exercises, the patient eventually uses the new movement patterns automatically in activities of daily living.

An awareness of a good posture in the standing position is essential. These patients tend to stand with a 'sway back', with an accentuated lumbar lordosis. This posture is corrected using active trunk muscle force to move from a position of solely passive support by spinal ligaments, which is thought to promote curve progression. Rotational breathing is then practised in the corrected posture.

Scoliosis

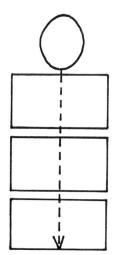

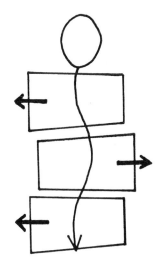

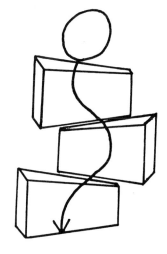

Fig. 2.70 Subdivision into three rectangular superimposed blocks.

Fig. 2.71 In scoliosis, three blocks deviate from the vertical axis → lateral shifting of spine.

Fig. 2.72 The three blocks develop 'wedge-like' form, and rotate against each other around the vertical axis. Ribs and spine follow these distortions. (Figs. 2.70–2.72 from C. Lehnert-Schroth, 1992. Introduction to the three-dimensional scoliosis treatment according to Schroth. *Physiotherapy,* **78**, 11, 813, with permission.)

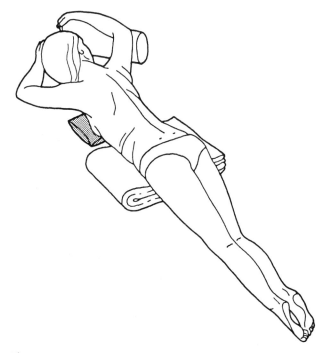

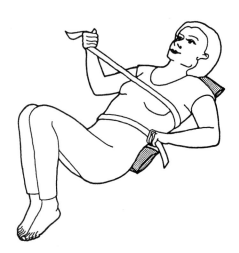

Fig. 2.69 Corrective exercises for scoliosis. Small, firm pads are strategically placed to stimulate the weak, overstretched muscles.

Fig. 2.73

Short leg syndrome

Many patients appear to have unequal leg lengths, most of which will have passed unnoticed. Shortening of less than 1 cm on one side is common. The whole leg may be shorter, in which case both knee and buttock creases will be lower on that side, or the femur alone may be shorter, in which case just the buttock crease will be lower (Fig. 2.74). Spinal deformities in the foot such as abnormal pronation of the subtalar joint, can give the appearance of shortening of the leg. It is impossible to measure leg length accurately using a tape measure over bony points, because torsion of the pelvis alters the position of its bony points.

Compensation for a short leg first occurs in the pelvis. Up to $\frac{1}{4}''$ can be taken up by the sacroiliac joint on the side of the longer leg. That ilium twists backwards, increasing the depth of the sulcus medial to the posterior superior iliac spine. If the discrepancy is small, the ilia may still appear level; if greater than $\frac{1}{2}''$, a lateral pelvic tilt occurs (Figs. 2.74, 2.75).

The usual compensation in the lumbar spine is a lateral curvature convex to the short leg side, sometimes with a lateral curve to the opposite side in the thoracic spine. The facets of the apophyseal joints on the concavity are compressed, which may be a factor in symptom production later in life, when age changes result in decreased height and further compression. On the side of the convexity, the annular fibres may be stretched, giving rise to symptoms earlier.

People with leg length inequality tend to stand asymmetrically, weight-bearing predominantly on the short leg side (Fig. 2.75). Repercussions on other joints may occur (*see* pp. 38–9) such as adaptive shortening in the hip on the side of the longer leg, reducing extension.

BACK CARE EMPHASIS

- The use of a heel raise should be considered in the following circumstances:

  1. If an obvious discrepancy is noticed in children or young adults whose spines are still flexible (In stiffer spines, a heel raise may result in an increase rather than a decrease of the curvature.)
  2. Where chronic pain persists arising from anywhere in the spine, despite treatment, in the presence of a short leg.

The short leg should be raised gradually and the pain response assessed. A rubber heel pad (about 1/8″) is inserted into the shoes and slippers of the short leg before advising a build-up of the heel of the shoe. For a week or two the patient may experience new stresses in his spine as it adjusts to the heel raise but, providing his original pain does not worsen, he should persist with the heel raise for at least three weeks and then be reassessed to see if a further slight increase might help. It is not always necessary to get the pelvis absolutely level for the raise to be successful and it is often inadvisable.

- If there is a structural deformity in the foot, an orthosis (as opposed to an arch support) may be necessary to correct faulty foot biomechanics.
- Posture re-education in standing may be necessary (*see* pp. 100–2).
- Iliopsoas stretches may be necessary on the side of the long leg (Fig. 5.14, p. 125).

Short Leg Syndrome

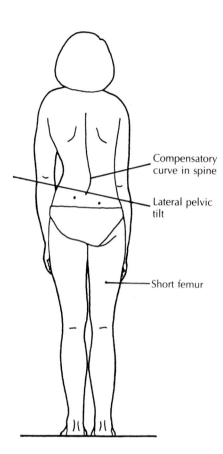

Compensatory
curve in spine

Lateral pelvic
tilt

Short femur

Fig. 2.74

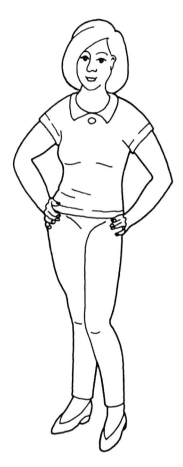

Fig. 2.75 Asymmetrical standing,
with more weight on
the short leg.

Forward Head Syndrome

In the normal head posture (Fig. 2.76), the apex of the lordotic cervical curve is at C4/5, but when the head is held forwards the curve changes: the lower cervical spine is held in flexion and, in order for the head to be positioned so that the person sees straight ahead, the lordosis is concentrated in the upper cervical spine. Depending on how far forwards the head is held, and the pathological state of the cervical spine, the apex may move as far cephalad as C1/2.

The forward head posture as depicted in Figs. 2.77, 2.78 is commonly associated with ageing. On closer inspection, however, it is evident that the deformity starts much earlier in life, and in many cases can be traced back to the teens. The positioning of the head more and more anterior to the centre of gravity happens so insidiously that it goes unnoticed by the patient and is, consequently, often well marked by the time symptoms occur.

This posture is usually associated with either a general increase in thoracic kyphosis (Fig. 2.77) or with a 'dowager's hump', i.e. a more localized kyphosis in the cervicothoracic area (Fig. 2.78).

It is difficult to state categorically an orderly sequence of events: does the deformity start with an increase in thoracic kyphosis or is this secondary to increased upper cervical extension? Most probably it varies in different individuals, and may occur simultaneously in others.

Causative activities include:

- Constant use of the arms in front of the body so that their weight, and forces imposed by them, pull on the lower cervical/thoracic spines, increasing the kyphosis. This includes most activities of daily living: when one considers the numbers of hours spent by women pushing buggies laden with babies and shopping, it is not difficult to envisage how the deformity may start, especially when fatigue sets in (Fig. 2.79).
- Hours spent working at a computer (Fig. 2.80)—now, of course, increasingly common in teenagers—with poor lighting and poor ergonomics. This may precipitate the forward head posture in an attempt to see the screen.
- This particular posture is also associated with a low self-esteem and depression. Anxiety begets muscular tension and one of the prime sites for this is in the neck extensors (Bannister, 1985).

Effect on cervical joints

Loss of normal anatomical alignment of the head and neck on the thoracic spine, together with some loss of mobility, may in time precipitate degenerative changes in the upper cervical synovial joints, and this has serious implications in terms of disturbed arthrokinetic impulses, which influence body posture. Abnormal stresses are also imposed on the cervicothoracic junction which is subjected to a torque force, and soft tissue thickening occurs in response. The weight-bearing facility of the motion segments is altered: some of the facet joints have to bear extra weight and the posterior annular fibres of the discs are compressed.

Forward Head Posture

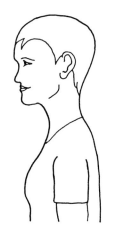

Fig. 2.76 Normal head posture.

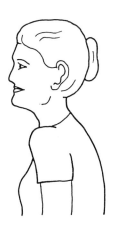

Fig. 2.77 Forward head posture: increase in thoracic kyphosis.

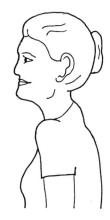

Fig. 2.78 Forward head posture: 'dowager's hump'.

Causes of forward head posture

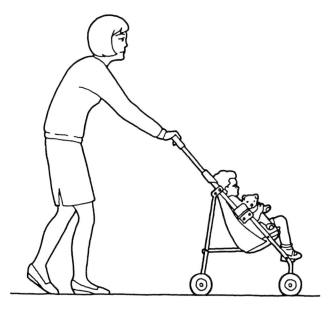

Fig. 2.79

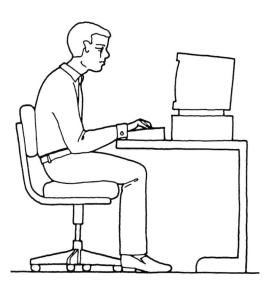

Fig. 2.80 Poor posture at computer. For correct posture, *see* Fig. 2.95.

Effect on muscles and soft tissues

There is shortening of the suboccipital muscles, levator scapulae, the upper fibres of trapezius and sternocleidomastoid with inhibition and weakness of the upper cervical flexors.

Overactivation of the suboccipital muscles and neck extensors occurs in the form of a sustained static contraction in order to keep the head level. As the centre of gravity of the head lies slightly anterior to the occipital condyles (Kapandji, 1974) even in the normal anatomical position, these muscles have to contract more than the flexors to maintain balance. The head weighs approximately 10 lb and the further forwards it is held, the heavier in effect it becomes, because a correspondingly greater force is required by the neck extensors to balance the weight of it (Fig. 2.81). Sustained traction on spinal nerves occurs in severe deformities.

Effects on movements

There is a loss of upper cervical flexion and lower cervical and upper thoracic extension. Rotation and lateral flexion in the whole of the cervical spine are both reduced because of the alteration in curvatures (Figs. 2.82, 2.83). Rotation tends to occur predominantly in the upper cervical spine. Further range is blocked lower down in the cervical spine because of the deformity and, therefore, increasing stiffness occurs.

Effects on other joints

This major alteration in posture may have far reaching effects on other joints. In some cases, the neck itself may be asymptomatic, but symptoms may arise because of the effects on other joints and tissues.

The position of the scapulae alters: shortening of the upper fibres of trapezius and levator scapulae cause some elevation and the increased thoracic convexity causes them to move into abduction. Muscles such as teres major consequently become shortened. Tightness of muscles leads to reciprocal inhibition of their antagonists (Janda, 1978), notably the lower fibres of trapezius and the rhomboids.

The altered position of the scapulae has a significant effect on shoulder mechanics (Donatelli, 1991). Shoulder elevation is reduced in this deformity.

Shortening of the suboccipital muscles has also been implicated as one of the causative factors in some temperomandibular joint disorders (Ayub *et al.*, 1984) by an alteration in the position of the occiput in a posteroinferior direction, which results in an upward and backward displacement of the mandible in the glenoid fossa.

Symptomatology

A variety of symptoms may eventually arise from this postural abnormality. Because it occurs insidiously, the joints and soft tissues first undergo a certain amount of painless deformation.

Headache is a common complaint; it is usually unilateral, but it can be bilateral. The sites of aching from the cervical spine are: frontal, orbital, temporal and occipital (Figs. 2.84, 2.85). Compression of upper cervical nerve roots is relatively rare; the ache is more often referred from upper cervical joints and soft tissues. Dizziness and feelings of nausea often accompany the headache. Generalized aching in the neck extensors together with pain where they insert into the occiput are associated with the 'tension' headache (Fig. 2.86).

Forward Head Posture

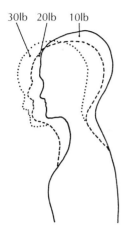

Fig. 2.81 Neck muscle activity increases the further forward the head is held.

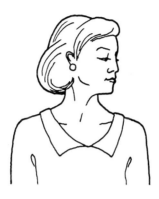

Fig. 2.82 Turning head: good posture.

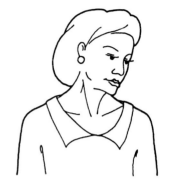

Fig. 2.83 Turning head: range of movement reduced with forward head posture.

'Cervical' headaches

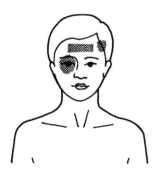

Fig. 2.84

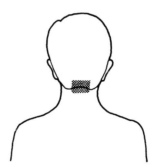

Fig. 2.85

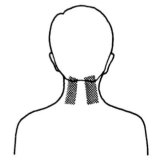

Fig. 2.86 'Muscle tension' headache.

Burning pain at the *cervicothoracic junction* can occur due to it having to take extra stress.

Muscular pain is usually bilateral in the upper fibres of trapezius due to sustained static contraction. It is possible that this may precipitate early spondylotic changes due to impaired movement.

Localized and referred pain from *apophyseal joints* can occur with increasing stiffness.

NECK CARE EMPHASIS

- *Explanation to patient* (Figs. 2.76–2.86).
  Many patients are initially unable to grasp the concept of bad posture causing trauma: so many people have poor posture but do not necessarily have symptoms. If symptoms do arise from superimposed trauma, they invariably take longer to correct if posture is poor.

  It is important to be realistic about what can be achieved in the way of correction. Asking the patient to reverse the posture (Fig. 2.87) and noting the ease with which he can do this is a good indicator of the length of time it will take to achieve results. Some patients cannot reverse their posture at a first attempt due to bony structural changes and/or soft tissue tightening, and may need individual mobilization treatment from the physiotherapist to assist. Although full correction will not be achieved in some patients, it is surprising how even a small improvement in posture brings relief of pain because of the improved mechanics. Often posture training is a long, slow process and the patient must be prepared to work at it!

  The patient must be absolutely clear about what he is asked to do and will often need many reminders. A convincing way of explaining correct head positioning is to use photographs of the patient showing his side view. Good head posture is more aesthetically pleasing and less ageing, which is an incentive to most people. It also makes the patient look taller. It helps if the patient places his fingers lightly on the neck extensors just distal to the occiput to feel the change in muscular tension as he moves his head back and forwards (Fig. 2.87). First in the forward head posture and then in a corrected position, the patient should be asked to rotate his head and neck and note the increase in range (Figs. 2.82, 2.83).

  Spinal posture as a whole should be considered (see correction of posture in the sitting position, pp. 88–9), the position of the head being adjusted in small stages. It feels wrong at first to the patient and, if overcorrected, he will not be able to hold the position. However, the use of exercises is invaluable in gaining an increase in the range of movement first.

- *Exercises*
  These should be practised three times a day to begin with to stretch the suboccipital muscles and then to strengthen the upper cervical flexors (Figs. 2.88, 2.89, 2.90), and to gain extension of the lower cervical spine (Fig. 2.91). Further exercises to stretch the pectoral muscles (Fig. 2.92) and strengthen the rhomboids may also be necessary.

Forward Head Syndrome

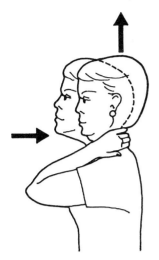

Fig. 2.87 Posture correction: feel change in muscle tone.

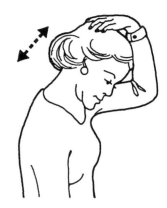

Fig. 2.89 Stretch for top of neck.

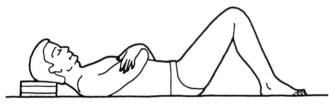

Fig. 2.88 Stretch for top of neck. Lie for 10 min, with head raised 4 cm. Gradually increase height of books.

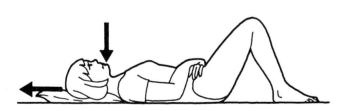

Fig. 2.90 Gravity-assisted exercise to stretch top of neck.

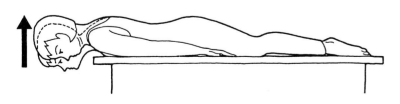

Fig. 2.91 Progression of Fig. 2.90 (gravity-resisted) to strengthen back of neck.

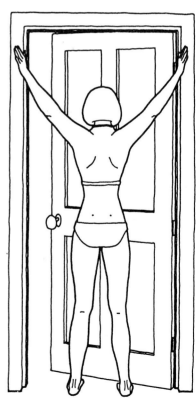

Fig. 2.92 Stretch for the tight pectoral muscles.

● *Analysis of particular aggravating factors* such as:

1. The *use of bifocals*, which encourage upper cervical extension when using the lower part of the lens.
2. Poor posture while *reading in bed* (Figs. 2.93, 2.94), or *working at a computer* (Fig. 2.80; *see* Fig. 2.95 for correct posture).
3. *Incorrect lifting technique:* the chin should be kept tucked in when lifting (Fig. 4.2, p. 109).
4. *Occupational hazards* — e.g. painting ceilings. Upper cervical extension should be interrupted frequently by upper cervical flexion stretches (Fig. 2.89).
5. *Swimming:* the breaststroke with the head out of the water (Fig. 2.96), the chin should be tucked in. If this is not possible, the patient should change to the crawl or backstroke.
6. *Muscle tension:* a degree of muscle spasm is always present in response to pain. However, where nervous tension is considered to be the main cause of the problem, the patient may be best advised to attend a good relaxation class or follow a particular method. Relaxing in a comfortable position with a heat pad moulded round the neck is a great help.

References

Abramson V., Roberts S. M., Wilson P. D. (1934). Relaxation of the pelvic joints in pregnancy. *Surg. Gynecol. Obstet.*, **58**, 595.

Adams M. A., Hutton W. C., Stott J. R. R. (1980). The resistance to flexion of the lumbar intervertebral joint. *Spine*, Vol. 5, 3, 245.

Adams M. A., Hutton W. C. (1983). The mechanical function of the lumbar apophyseal joints. *Spine*, **8**, 3, 327.

Adams M. A., Hutton W. C. (1985). Gradual disc prolapse. *Spine*, **10**, 6, 524.

Adams M. A., Dolan P., Hutton W. C. (1987). Diurnal variations in the stresses on the lumbar spine. *Spine*, **12**, 2, 130.

Ansell B. M. (1972). Hypermobility of joints. *Mod. Trends Orthop.*, **6**, 419.

Ayub E., Glasheen-Wray M., Kraus S. (1984). Head posture: a case study of the effects on the rest position of the mandible. *J. Orthop. Sports Phys. Ther.*, 5, 179.

Bannister R. (1985). *Brain's Clinical Neurology*. 64th edn. London: Oxford University Press.

Beighton P., Grahame R., Bird H. (1983). *Hypermobility of Joints*, Berlin, Heidelberg: Springer-Verlag.

Bird H. A., Tribe C. R., Bacon P. A. (1978). Joint hypermobility leading to osteoarthrosis and chondrocalcinosis. *Ann. Rheum. Dis.*, **37**, 203.

Dale W. D., Baer E., Keller A. *et al.* (1972). On the ultrastructure of mammalian tendon. *Experientia*, **28**, 1293.

Dixon A. St. J. (1986), Osteoporosis – an unheeded epidemic. *Practitioner*, **230**, 363.

Donatelli R. A., ed. (1991). *Clinics in Physical Therapy: Physical Therapy of the Shoulder*, 2nd edn. New York, Edinburgh, London, Melbourne: Churchill Livingstone.

Dunlop R. B., Adams M. A., Hutton W. C. (1984). Disc space narrowing and the lumbar facet joints. *J. Bone Jt. Surg.*, **66–B**, 5, 706.

Frank C., Amiel D., Woo S. L-Y. (1985). Normal ligament properties and ligament healing. *Clin. Orthopaed. & Rel. Res.*, **196**, 15.

Forward head syndrome

Reading in Bed

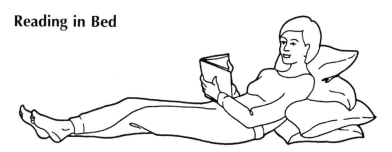

Fig. 2.93 Strain on neck.

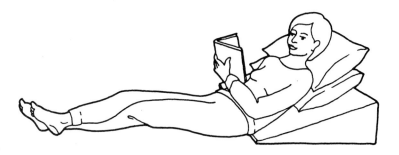

Fig. 2.94 Improved neck posture.

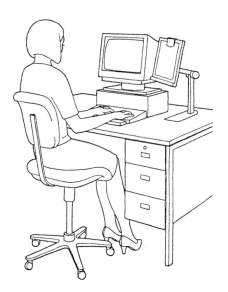

Fig. 2.95 Correct posture at VDU.

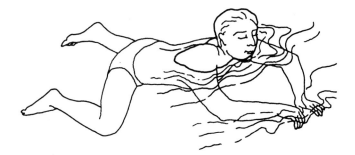

Fig. 2.96 Strain on neck. Chin should be tucked in during breaststroke.

Grahame R., Edwards J. C., Pitcher D. *et al.* (1981). A clinical and echocardiographic study of patients with the hypermobility syndrome. *Ann. Rheum. Dis.*, **40**, 541.

Harris H., Joseph J. (1949). Variation in extension of the metacarpophalangeal and interphalangeal joints of the thumb. *J. Bone Jt. Surg.* (Br.), **31**, 4, 547.

Hayne C. R. (1987). *Total Back Care*, London, Melbourne: J. M. Dent.

Janda V. (1978). Muscles, motor regulation and back problems, 27. In *The Neurologic Mechanisms in Manipulative Therapy* (Korr I. R., ed.). New York: Plenum.

Kapandji I. A. (1974). *The Physiology of the Joints, 3, The Trunk and the Vertebral Column*, Edinburgh: Churchill Livingstone.

Kirk J. A., Ansell B. M., Bywaters E. G. L. (1967). The hypermobility syndrome. *Ann. Rheum. Dis.*, 26, 419.

Krolner B., Toft B., Nielson S. P. *et al.* (1983). Physical exercise as prophylaxis against involutional vertebral bone loss: a controlled trial. *Clin. Sci.*, **64**, 541.

Lindblom K. (1957). Intervertebral disc degeneration considered as a pressure atrophy. *J. Bone Joint Surg.*, **39A**, 933.

Malinsky J. (1959). The ontogenetic development of nerve terminations in the intervertebral discs of man. *Acta Anat.*, **38**, 96.

Nachemson A. (1976). The lumbar spine: an orthopaedic challenge. *Spine*, **1**, 59.

Newman P. H. (1968). 'The spine, the wood and the trees'. *Proc. Roy. Soc. Med.*, **61**, 35.

Oliver J., Middleditch A. (1991). *Functional Anatomy of the Spine*. Oxford: Butterworth Heinemann.

Postacchini F., Lami R., Pugliese O. (1988). Familial predisposition to discogenic low-back pain. An epidemiologic and immunogenetic study. *Spine*, **13**, 12, 1403.

Rissanen P. M. (1960). The surgical anatomy and pathology of the supraspinous and interspinous ligaments of the lumbar spine with special reference to ligament ruptures. *Acta Orthop. Scand.*, (Suppl), 46.

Scheuermann H. (1921). Zur Röentgensymptomatologie der juvelinen Osteochondritis Dorsi. *Z. Orthop. Chir.*, **41**, 305.

Stoddard A. (1983). *Manual of Osteopathic Practice*, 2nd edn. London: Hutchinson.

Troup J. D. G. (1979). Biomechanics of the vertebral column. *Physiotherapy*, **65**, 8, 239.

Wyke B. (1976). Neurological aspects of low back pain. In *The Lumbar Spine and Back Pain* (Jayson M. I. V., ed.) London: Sector Publishing.

Further Reading

Lehnert-Schroth C. (1992). Introduction to the three-dimensional scoliosis treatment according to Schroth. *Physiotherapy*, **78**, 11, 810.

Weiss H. R. (1992). The progression of idiopathic scoliosis under the influence of a physiotherapy rehabilitation programme. *Physiotherapy*, **78**, 11, 815.

3
Posture

Good posture is the attitude a person assumes, using the minimum amount of muscular effort and, at the same time, protecting the supporting structures against trauma.

There are considerable variations between individuals in the amount of muscular effort used when performing identical tasks (Lundervold, 1951). Some people use a degree of muscular effort which is out of all proportion to the end it achieves. In habitually tense or rigid postures, the muscles exert unnecessarily high pressures over the joints and may well precipitate early degenerative changes in them. Conversely, a common cause of ligamentous strains is the faulty posture which involves the use of hardly any muscle work at all: instead of using his postural muscles for support, the person (frequently hypermobile, *see* p. 24) maintains the posture by 'hanging on his ligaments' (*see* Fig. 2.47).

Prolonged asymmetrical postures may also lead to structural changes by causing fibroblasts in the muscles to multiply along the lines of stress and produce more collagen (Editorial, 1979). These extra collagen fibres take up space in the connective tissue of the muscles and start to encroach on the space normally occupied by nerves, blood and lymphatic vessels. The muscle loses some elasticity and may become painful when required to do work, especially if used statically. In the long term, the collagen begins to replace the active fibres of the muscle. Clinically, similar changes are apparent in the soft tissues of a scoliotic spine that has stiffened up.

Correct spinal balance and posture is a prerequisite to efficient use of the limbs. Postural deviations such as the forward head posture and the lordotic low back may have far reaching consequences on other joints such as (a) the shoulders and temperomandibular joints (*see* p. 54) and (b) the hips, knees and feet.

Postural sensation is dependent on joint, cutaneous and myotatic (muscle spindle) mechanoreceptors (Wyke, 1981), of which there is a particularly abundant supply in the upper cervical spine. Degenerative disease affecting for instance the apophyseal joints, impairs postural and kinaesthetic sensations. There are many other causes of faulty posture, and these are considered in the following pages, together with suggestions on how to correct them.

Lying

Approximately one-third of our lives is spent in bed, so the effect of a particular bed and the position/s we lie in is, therefore, a very relevant consideration. Patients need some explanation, however, as to what constitutes a 'good' bed. They often think that an 'orthopaedic' bed is the best type, falling prey to advertising loopholes that allow any rock-hard bed, unsuitable for most people, to be called 'orthopaedic'. A bed is an expensive item and most people can ill afford to make a mistake when buying one. To judge a bed's merits by lying on it for a few minutes in the shop is inadequate because, if one is tired from walking around, any bed will seem comfortable for such a short period of time.

When is the bed likely to be contributing to the patient's symptoms? The answer may appear to be obvious, but it is surprising how seemingly poor beds may not be an aggravating factor to the patient's problem. The therapist should consider giving advice concerning the bed:

- *If the patient's symptoms wake him during the night*: This *could* indicate that the bed is unsuitable or it could be caused by the patient's lying position. Also, the pathology needs to be considered: inflammatory joint conditions often worsen with rest, and most acute lesions are aggravated by movements such as turning over in bed. Patients with highly irritable lesions are usually more comfortable lying on a very firm support that gives them more control over movements. However, as the patient's back improves, this very firm support, which was so useful in the acute stage, may prove to be too unresilient for him.
- *If the patient has symptoms on waking in the morning*: Again, this may not necessarily be the fault of the bed; symptoms felt on waking are often the result of the previous day's activities.
- *If the bed seems to be a potential source of trouble*: If the patient's bed is blatantly lumpy and unsuitable, even though it is not contributing to his present symptoms, some simple guidelines regarding future choice of beds could be given after dealing with the immediate priorities.

Temporary measures to improve the bed

To make the bed firmer:

A sheet of 1.5 cm or (if symptoms are severe) 2 cm chipboard can be placed between base and mattress, preferably covering the whole area of the base. (Fig. 3.1).

A mattress placed on the floor (*not* by the patient!) can be a useful temporary measure, but only if getting up and down from the floor is not too traumatic for him. It is inadvisable to adopt this measure on the first night after a spinal injury, especially if the patient lives alone, as symptoms often increase during the first night and he may find himself unable to get up unaided.

To make the bed softer:

A duvet, sleeping bag or a 5 cm sheet of foam rubber placed over a too-hard mattress can be a great improvement (Fig. 3.2).

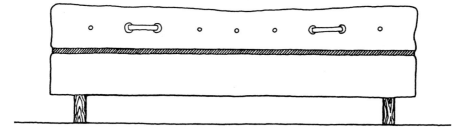

Fig. 3.1 To make bed firmer: place 1.5 cm chipboard between base and mattress.

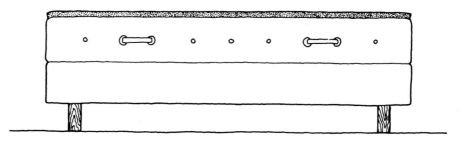

Fig. 3.2 To make bed softer: place 5 cm sheet of foam rubber or a duvet over mattress.

Guidelines on choosing a bed

It is unwise to recommend a particular make of bed to the patient; he must make the final choice himself. First, sleeping in a different bed, e.g. a spare bed in the house or at a friend's, will give the patient some idea as to which type of surface will suit him. A good bed should support the natural curves of the spine in their anatomical position and, therefore, the person's weight has to be taken into account. A lighter person's spine will conform in a different manner to that of a heavier person when lying on the same type of mattress.

General guidelines:

The base is just as important as the mattress, and it should be firm: wooden slats, for example, provide this type of base.
The mattress. A medium-firm mattress is often most suitable for patients who, despite adequate mobilization and exercise, have stiff spines, or those with marked curves such as kyphosis or kyphoscoliosis. This type of mattress accommodates the hip and shoulder in the side-lying position. Very firm mattresses such as those made from thick foam rubber are occasionally preferred, e.g. by patients with very mobile spines. Older people often find that a softer, more yielding mattress suits them, as do patients with chronic femoral nerve lesions. In the final analysis, comfort should be the deciding factor.
Double beds. A double bed should be at least 5 ft wide to allow freedom of movement for each person. If there is a marked difference in the weight—and preference—of those using the bed, two single beds which zip up the middle, with a mattress to suit each person is one solution.

Sleeping positions

The position/s patients adopt in bed can either aggravate or ease back and neck pain. A position which is initially comfortable may cause pain if held for a long time (e.g. the 'fetal' position in patients with acute disc pathology). On the whole, positions which place the joints at the end of any range should be avoided unless there is no other choice of a pain-relieving position.

The **prone-lying position** (Fig. 3.3) encourages inner range lumbar extension which causes bony contact between the inferior articular facets of the apophyseal joints and the laminae below, and stresses these joints at the end of their range. If this is the *only* position in which pain is relieved, then of course the patient should use it, but otherwise he should be discouraged from sleeping in it. The back can become 'locked' in this position, and the patient then has difficulty getting out of it. The neck also suffers (*see* p. 66). There is often great reluctance on the part of patients to stop sleeping prone, and they will argue that they end up prone even if they start off in another position. However, it is surprising how even the subconscious mind can be trained, if the patient has the will and sees the reason for it. As a compromise, the extreme prone-lying position can be modified by flexing one hip and knee and raising one arm (Fig. 3.4). If the patient has pain on lying down, he should at least start the night in one of the resting positions shown in Figs 3.5–7.

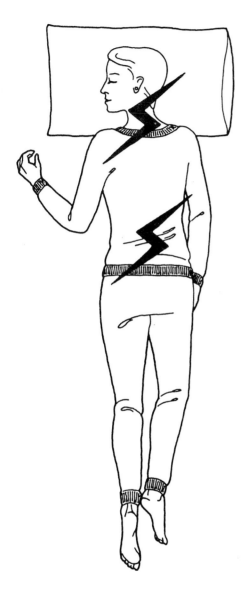

Fig. 3.3 The prone-lying position places joints at the end of their range.

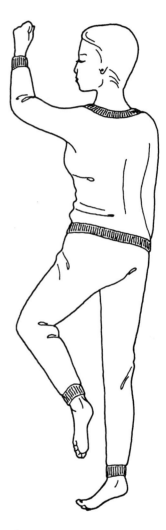

Fig. 3.4 Modified prone-lying position.

Patients with back pain provoked by activities of daily living benefit from taking the weight off their backs for 20 minutes or so at least once a day, depending on how severe the pain is. After lunch is a good time, to prevent a buildup of symptoms. A heat pad behind the lower spine to aid muscle relaxation may also help, and gives the patient the feeling that he is treating his back rather than just having a rest.

Comfortable resting positions vary from patient to patient, principally depending on the pathological condition and its state of irritability. There is no point lying in any position that eventually worsens the pathology, e.g. sometimes patients with acute disc pathology find that the fetal position temporarily relieves symptoms, but later (because this position allows more posterior movement of the nucleus) considerably worsens them.

If flexion in standing aggravates symptoms, the patient will invariably be more comfortable with the lumbar spine in either neutral or in some degree of extension. The positions shown in Figs. 3.5–3.9 will often help.

Conversely, patients whose symptoms are relieved by flexion (e.g. those with arthrosis in the lumbar spine) may obtain relief in one of the positions shown in Figs. 3.10–3.12.

In the side-lying position, pillows of appropriate thickness should fill the gap between the point of the shoulder and the neck (Fig. 3.13) to keep the cervical spine in a neutral position. A small pillow in the waist can prevent lateral flexion in the lumbar spine (Fig. 3.14). This is more applicable to women with large hips and a small waist. One or two pillows between the knees can prevent torsion strains in the lumbar area (Fig. 3.15).

In the acute stage of sciatica caused by pathology in the disc, it is sometimes difficult to find a comfortable resting position. Those shown in Figs. 3.4 and 3.11 often give some relief. One small pillow under the head or, ideally, none at all should be used, to avoid neuromeningeal tension.

Neck comfort

A good neck posture during sleep rates highly in the prevention of neck disorders. It is very difficult to get a good night's sleep if the neck is unsuitably supported. One sleeping position that is a frequent cause of symptoms arising from the neck, e.g. headache, dizziness, paraesthesia in the arm, is prone-lying (*see also* p. 64). In this position, the cervical spine is more or less at the end of its rotation range, compressing the joints on the side to which the head is rotated and stretching those on the opposite side. Similar trauma is caused to the nerve roots. Often patients who have previously had hypermobile necks choose this position, but it should be discouraged because even if treatment is helping the patient's neck, it will rarely get better if they continue to sleep prone.

Comfortable resting positions

If pain is made worse by bending:

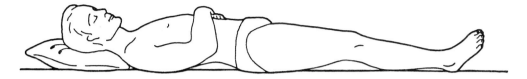

Fig. 3.5 Slightly arch low back.

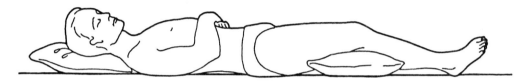

Fig. 3.6 Pillow placed under knees reduces arch.

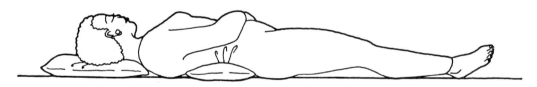

Fig. 3.7 Pillow placed in waist increases arch.

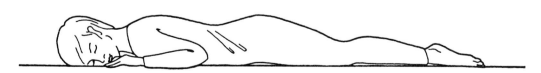

Fig. 3.8 Prone-lying is useful for short periods only.
Patient must be able to get out of this position.

Comfortable resting positions

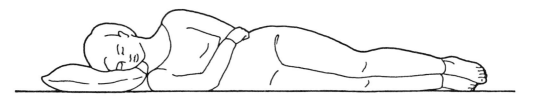

Fig. 3.9   Neutral.

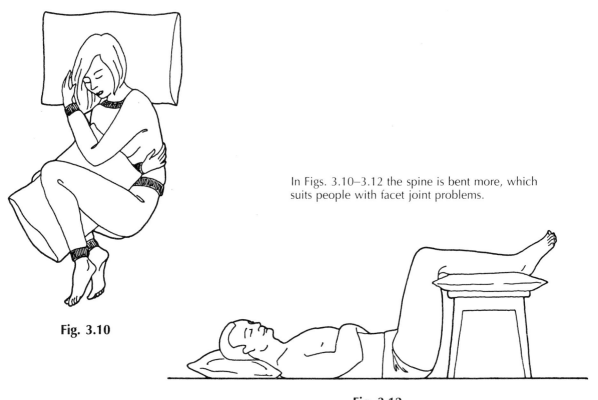

Fig. 3.10

In Figs. 3.10–3.12 the spine is bent more, which suits people with facet joint problems.

Fig. 3.12

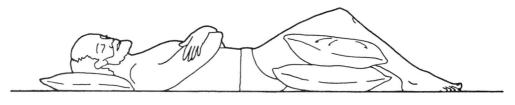

Fig. 3.11

Comfortable resting positions

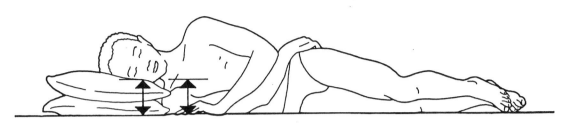

Fig. 3.13 Two pillows may be needed if shoulders are broad.

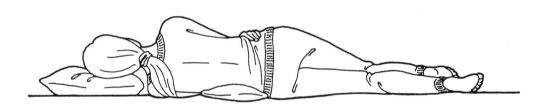

Fig. 3.14 Pillow in waist prevents side-bending.

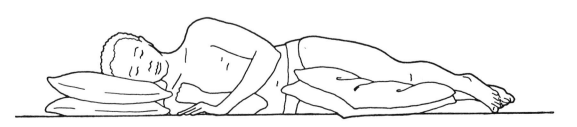

Fig. 3.15 Pillows between knees prevent spine rotating.

Types of pillows

Nowadays a wide range of pillows is available: down, feather, foam chips and moulded foam to name but a few. A down pillow is easy to tuck into the neck to give support where it is needed and is often preferred, at least as a top pillow. Price, however, is sometimes prohibitive. Feather pillows vary a lot. The feathers may be naturally curly or they may be artificially curled; the latter type becomes less supportive more quickly as the feathers uncurl. A useful test to see if a pillow has any life left in it is punching it in the middle to see if it springs back into shape. Foam may have to be used by the allergic types, but often foam chips aggravate an acute neck as they cause movement when it may not be desirable. There are many excellent moulded foam pillows available, but the patient should always try one out first before buying it and not be misled by advertising claims.

Number of pillows

It is difficult to advise patients as to the exact number of pillows to use at home without actually seeing what pillows he has, because one new pillow may give the same support as two old ones. On the whole, the general principle of supporting the neck in its neutral position applies. In the side-lying position, therefore, shoulder width largely determines the number of pillows needed (Fig. 3.13).

In supine, flexion of the neck should generally be avoided except:

1. in the presence of a low cervical nerve root problem where say, three pillows may be necessary to relieve pressure on the nerve root (Fig. 3.16).
2. where a *fixed* flexion deformity exists, e.g. in elderly people. This has to be accommodated with pillows, otherwise relaxation is impossible.

In the presence of cardiac, respiratory problems or other medical conditions such as hiatus hernia, raising the head end of the bed on blocks (Fig. 3.17) may be more comfortable than putting lots of pillows under the head. If this is not possible (e.g. in a double bed), the pillows should be placed so as to avoid excessive neck flexion.

Temporary measures to support the acute neck

1. A foam roll placed inside the pillow case (Fig. 3.18) to support the cervical spine can give relief to those patients whose symptoms are aggravated by neck flexion.
2. Make a 'butterfly' pillow: take a pillow out of its case, twist it round in the middle and put it back in its case (Fig. 3.19). The 'butterfly' pillow can either be used as the only pillow or as the top pillow, depending on comfort. It helps to prevent the head rolling into rotation or lateral flexion.
3. Sandbags placed under each side of the pillow have a similar effect. In acute nerve root lesions, pillows strategically placed relieve tension on the nerve roots, e.g. for C5 lesions, one or two pillows under the affected arm (Fig. 3.20).

Comfortable positions to relieve 'nerve' pain in arm

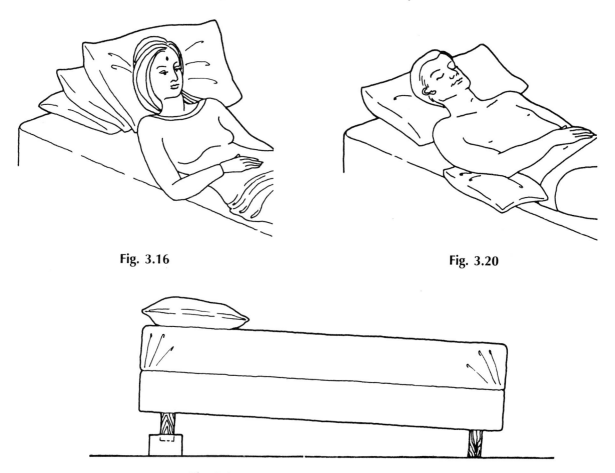

Fig. 3.16   **Fig. 3.20**

Fig. 3.17   For patients who are unable to lie flat:
raising the head of the bed prevents neck
strain caused by using too many pillows.

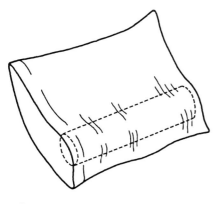

Fig. 3.18   Foam roll inside pillow
case to support neck.

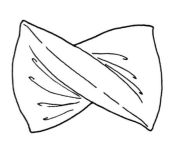

Fig. 3.19   A 'butterfly'
pillow.

Bedmaking

The more widespread use of duvets as opposed to blankets and sheets has saved many a back. For those who are reluctant to use duvets, the tucking in of the bedclothes under the mattress is the commonest cause of lumbar stress.

If this is done in combination with flexion, even greater stress is imposed. It is better to kneel to do this, and brace the abdomen to protect the lumbar spine (Fig. 3.21). As, usually, the bed is made first thing in the morning, this is another 'danger time' (*see* p. 30) for patients with discogenic pathology, and bedmaking might be more sensibly left until later in the day.

Getting in and out of bed

To keep the spine in as neutral a position as possible, the patient should:

- flex hips and knees into the crook-lying position;
- roll onto side all in one piece;
- put lower legs over the side of the bed;
- push with arms into the sitting position (Figs. 3.22–3.24).

The reverse procedure should be used for getting into bed.

However, with acute spinal lesions, the patient should be allowed to use his own method, however slow and unorthodox it may appear, if he has found one that is less painful than that described above. A chair by the bedside is a useful support. Sometimes patients find that first turning over into the prone position (Fig. 3.25) and then pushing with the arms to extend the lumbar spine as they get out of bed is less stressful.

Travelling

Hotel beds are notoriously uncomfortable, and, coupled with the hours spent in a car and carrying luggage, can be a potential hazard. Advance requests when the room booking is made, for a firm bed or a board under the mattress are often met or, of course, if space permits the mattress could be placed on the floor as a last resort.

Bedrest

The value of bedrest for selected patients cannot be overstated. For maximum beneficial effect, however, it must be used at the crucial time, i.e. in the acute stage of a lesion rather than in the chronic stage, and the patient should be gradually weaned off it. There is little sense in sentencing a patient to three weeks' bedrest and then telling him to go straight back to work. A few days' bedrest can often settle a lesion which would otherwise at best take three weeks to resolve and, at worst, progress to nerve root involvement.

Therapists working in an out-patients department may never have had the opportunity to see a really acute back. In the main, their patients walk into the department. Even if in pain, the patient has managed to get there. In the acute stage of severe back pain, the patient can hardly move, let alone leave the house, and he is far better managed at home. Even if he is successfully treated in an out-patient department, he still has to get home, and often the journey back, if he has to sit, completely negates the value of the treatment.

Getting out of bed
keeping spine in neutral position

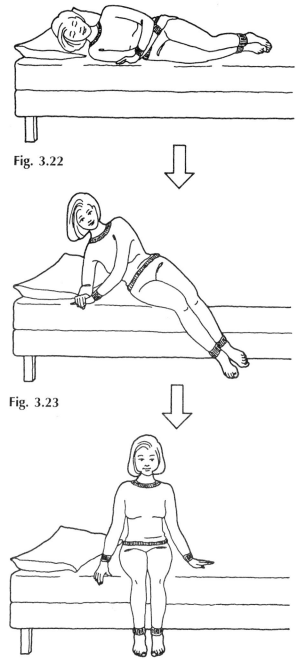

Fig. 3.22

Fig. 3.23

Fig. 3.24

Reverse procedure for
getting into bed

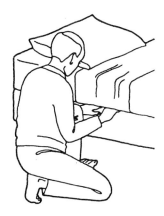

Fig. 3.21 Bedmaking: kneel and brace tummy muscles.

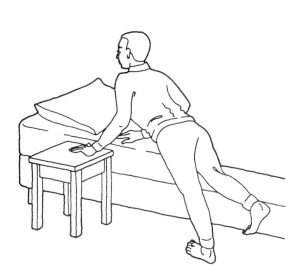

Fig. 3.25 Getting out of bed from the prone position is easier for some people.

Just as any peripheral musculoskeletal lesion benefits from rest in the acute stage, so does the spine. Depending on the severity of the lesion, the necessary amount of rest will vary accordingly. If pain is not too severe, a corset will provide some rest for the lumbar spine, remind the patient not to bend and, if tightly fitting, will reduce intradiscal pressure. It enables the patient to be ambulant. If the pain is more severe, the patient may also have to lie down in a comfortable resting position several times a day. Complete 24-hours a day bedrest should be reserved for those patients with highly irritable lesions when symptoms are aggravated by the slightest movement. Patients with severe discogenic disorders may obtain little relief even on bedrest for the first three days, and this is where firm guidance is necessary to reassure them that bedrest is still the best choice. It is often unnecessary for the patient to lie supine all the time—indeed, sometimes this can be the worst position for pain relief. Ideally, the patient needs at least two positions in which to lie (*see* pp. 64–9 for comfortable resting positions), and to be able to move from one to the other. Any position, no matter how comfortable it is to start with, becomes intolerable after a while. The position shown in Fig. 3.26 should be avoided.

Regular assessment by the therapist will confirm whether or not the lesion is improving. Even minor improvements in the patient's condition, e.g. ability to turn over in bed when previously this movement may have provoked pain, is a positive sign that the lesion is subsiding provided, of course, that pain has not been replaced by positive neurological signs.

Complete 24-hour a day bedrest strictly means that the patient should use bedpans instead of going to the toilet, but this is often far more traumatic than using crutches or crawling to get to the toilet, and is impractical for patients living on their own. Patients nearly always prefer to have this small vestige of independence. Whichever method results in less after-effects should be chosen.

Bedrest is difficult for most people: it is *always* inconvenient. Patients may regard it as a non-treatment and want 'action', e.g. manipulation. The needs of the patient's job and family weigh heavily on him and, if help cannot be provided by family, friends or neighbours, patients sometimes have to be admitted to hospital for bedrest. This is hardly cost-effective, and other assistance, e.g. home helps, should be considered first. Bedrest is mentally trying for most people, and this is one of the reasons why it is often cut short. The patient should be provided with reading material or games and have access to music, radio, television, etc., but his position when, for instance, writing, should not be such as to strain his back. Half-sitting should be discouraged. It helps the patient to keep to a light diet so that he avoids straining at faeces.

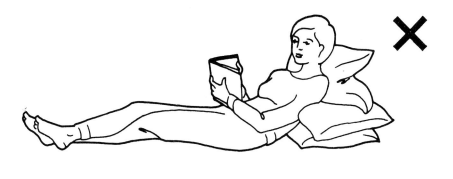

Fig. 3.26

Gentle exercising, though not those which produce symptoms, can help to make the patient feel he is participating in a positive way to his recovery. The exercises need not necessarily be for the back unless a pain-relieving one can be found; gentle quadriceps tightening, foot circling, etc., are useful.

Activities should be introduced as and when the patient is able to perform them without aggravating the condition, and not at a pre-selected time. As soon as he can stand comfortably for a few minutes without prolonged after-effects, he should be encouraged to do so, and this should be attempted periodically. Sitting is usually the most painful position and should be used cautiously. Intradiscal pressure is increased when sitting (*see* p. 31), and patients should only sit for a minute or two to begin with and then assess its after-effects before progressing. For more details on sitting *see* pp. 76–91. Usually patients with acute backs prefer to sit high rather than low to avoid lumbar flexion, with a lumbar support and, perhaps, a wedge to keep the pelvis tilted forwards. As soon as discomfort is felt, he should lie down again or walk around. Gradually, the extent of time that the patient can tolerate each activity will increase, and the spine is thus allowed to heal without further trauma occurring.

When is bedrest not useful?

Further bedrest is unlikely to help if, after an acute episode of spinal pain when bedrest has been strictly adhered to for three weeks, there is no sign whatever of improvement. This is relatively rare.

Spinal pain caused by stiffness is made worse by bedrest—indeed, it only perpetuates the problem.

Sitting

Any posture that is sustained has unhealthy implications for the body (*see* pp. xiii–iv). The prolonged sitting posture is undoubtedly the most unhealthy, and one of the most common complaints of people with back pain is inability to sit in comfort, with difficulty in straightening the back on rising. In industrialized countries, the tendency is for people to sit during most of the day; even in many schools, children are expected to sit most of the time.

Whenever, over the years, any posture is used for long periods the body's structures adapt to that position—tissues on the concavities shorten while those on the convexities lengthen, and a state of muscle imbalance occurs (Janda, 1988). Because of this, the habitual sitting posture adopted by each individual, when used extensively, also influences other postures, e.g. the standing posture. It is important, therefore, that we consider first what happens in sitting postures and, secondly, how we can break up these prolonged periods of a relatively static posture.

What happens when we sit?

We can sit in a wide variety of positions, each of which has a different effect on the spine. The position most frequently analysed is that of unsupported sitting on a horizontal surface with a trunk/thigh angle of 90° (the right-angled sitting posture) (Fig. 3.27). In this position:

1. The pelvis is tilted backwards, flattening the lumbar lordosis. The 90° trunk/thigh angle represents 60° hip flexion and 30° lumbar flexion (Schoberth, 1962), most of which takes place at the two lowest lumbar levels.
2. Intradiscal pressure is higher than in standing (Fig. 2.26, p. 31) due to the compressive effect of psoas major (Keagy *et al.*, 1966), flexion of the motion segment (Nachemson, 1965), and the fact that weight is shifted from the apophyseal joints more onto the discs.
3. Intradiscal pressure can be reduced to some extent by the sitter arching the low back in this position.
4. Static muscle work is needed to maintain this position as there is no outside spinal support.

Even when people are trained in correct posture, this unsupported position cannot be tolerated for long: the static contraction of the erectores spinae is tiring and undesirable, and the position is unstable. The body attempts to stabilize itself in a number of unsatisfactory ways:

1. By collapsing into a slouched position (Fig. 3.28).
2. The strain is then taken by stretched ligaments (p. 20) which eventually register pain, and there is a further rise in intradiscal pressure. In order to hold the head upright, there is a marked increase in muscle activity in the upper fibres of trapezius and deep neck extensors.
3. To obtain further stability, the sitter often crosses his legs (Fig. 3.29). The hip of the upper leg 'locks' near the end of the range of flexion-adduction, and the pelvis rotates slightly to the opposite side, taking with it the lower lumbar spine. Muscles fatigue faster in asymmetrical sitting postures, and further adjustments are soon required.

Effects of unsupported sitting

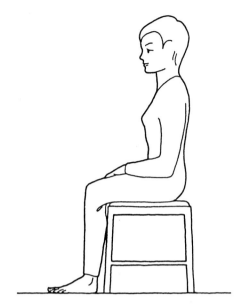

Fig. 3.27 With no spinal support, static muscle work is needed to maintain this right-angled position.

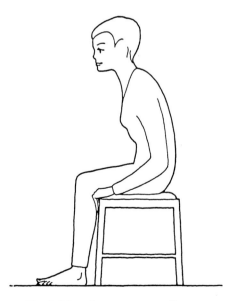

Fig. 3.28 The sitter soon collapses into a slouched position, stretching ligaments.

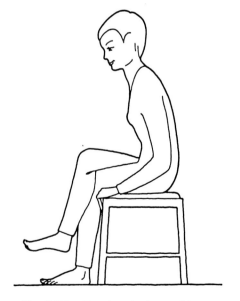

Fig. 3.29 Crossing the legs achieves further stability. The back is now effectively locked.

Choosing a suitable chair

The purpose for which a chair is being used has to be considered; one which is comfortable for relaxation purposes would not suit a person working at a VDU. The criteria are that the sitter's joints are adequately stabilized so that he is comfortable both in the chair and on rising from it. This will usually mean that the joints are near their middle-range with static muscle work kept to a minimum.

Different features in chair design can either reduce or increase muscle activity and intradiscal pressure. People often have fixed ideas about what constitutes a good chair, and we should offer them guidelines concerning individual features of chairs that need to be considered, as follows:

Backrest

A backrest is essential to provide stability for the sitter. A vertical backrest provides virtually no support because it prevents the sitter from leaning backwards. The tendency is for the sitter to slide his buttocks forwards to obtain support (Fig. 3.30). When the backrest is inclined backwards (Fig. 3.31), muscle activity in the back extensors and intradiscal pressure are reduced. For relaxation purposes, a backwardly inclined backrest is ideal, but to prevent the buttocks sliding forwards on the seat (Fig. 3.32), the thighs need to be raised (Fig. 3.33). In a working situation, where the sitter has to lean forwards over a desk, it is periodically useful for him to lean backwards to rest his back muscles and reduce intradiscal pressure and, for this reason, an adjustable backrest is invaluable.

Lumbar support

The use of a lumbar support has a marked influence on the degree of lumbar lordosis and, therefore, on spinal posture as a whole. The benefits of using a lumbar support are achieved when the sitter supports his spine on a backrest which is inclined backwards.

Any lumbar support which encourages more extension in the lumbar spine will correspondingly reduce intradiscal pressure. The curvature of the lumbar spine when using a support with a depth of 4 cm resembles closely that in the standing posture (Andersson *et al.*, 1979). However, the lumbar spine should not be held at the end of its range of extension, so for individuals with a naturally flat back, a very deep lumbar support would be uncomfortable. Patients appreciate being given the opportunity to try out different lumbar supports in the chair or car seat that they are using to see which one they prefer. The support should be placed where the patient finds it comfortable, which may be very low in the back behind the sacrum or higher depending on comfort. In the acute stage of a spinal lesion, the patient will often prefer more lumbar support than later on. To consider any permanent adjustments in the acute stage is, therefore, inadvisable.

Patients with the type of back which is more comfortable in flexion, e.g. those with arthrosis, spinal stenosis or spondylolisthesis, often dislike sitting with their back arched, and are often more comfortable in a carseat.

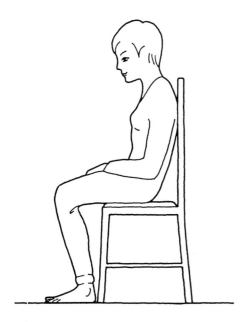

Fig. 3.30 A vertical backrest provides inadequate support.

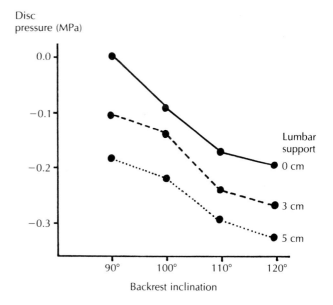

Fig. 3.31 The effect of backrest inclination and lumbar support on intradiscal pressure. (Adapted from A. Nachemson, 1976. The lumbar spine: an orthopaedic challenge. *Spine,* **1,** 59–71.)

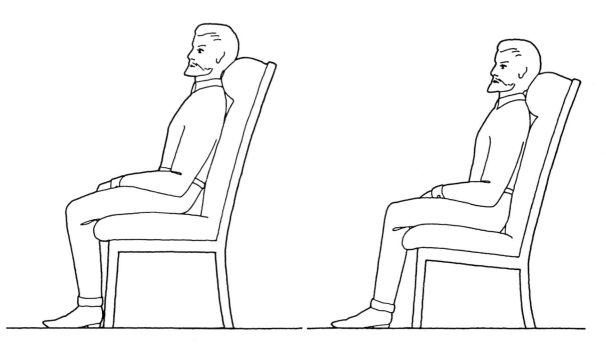

Fig. 3.32 Without a footrest, the buttocks slide forwards.

Fig. 3.33 When the backrest is inclined backwards, the thighs need to be raised.

Angle of seat
(Figs. 3.34–3.36)

The angle of the seat in relation to the horizontal affects the trunk/thigh angulation. A seat which slopes backwards decreases the angle and encourages more lumbar flexion than one which slopes forwards. This is particularly relevant for the person who is writing at a desk. School children are often scolded for leaning forward on their chairs (Fig. 6.1, p. 135) where this is an attempt to slope the seat forwards to get nearer to their work while reducing lumbar flexion. The exact amount of forward tilt may be critical for the comfort of the patient. To test whether he would be more comfortable with his seat sloping forwards, the rear legs of the patient's seat can be raised on blocks (Fig. 3.37), or wedges with varying heights can be placed on the seat (Fig. 3.38).* Consideration may also have to be given to the lumbar support, the position of which will be automatically altered by any adjustment to the seat angle.

It is perhaps unwise to recommend or condemn any particular item of furniture; rather the patient, with guidance, should try it out for himself. The kneeling stool (Fig. 3.39) has attracted considerable interest, and we are often asked our opinions regarding its suitability for patients. It has its advantages and disadvantages. Body weight is taken through the forward tilted seat and the knees are supported on a knee pad. This has the effect of reducing lumbar intradiscal pressure. Patients in the acute stage of disc and ligamentous problems can sometimes sit for a short period on this stool, whereas they are unable to sit on a horizontal surface. However, there is no back support, which means that a sustained muscular contraction is required to maintain the upright position unless further support, e.g. arm support, is used. Some patients find that their knees cannot tolerate the kneeling position; in particular, older people find this to be so. Therefore, for prolonged periods the kneeling stool has significant disdavantages for some patients, but it undoubtedly has its uses for some acute backs for short periods.

Firmness of seat

A soft surface, such as that of a settee, where the sitter sinks into a concavity, causes the hips to rotate internally, exposing the sciatic nerve to pressure laterally. Usually a firm, rather than a hard, support is more comfortable with a 'waterfall' front edge (*see* Fig. 3.44) to prevent pressure behind the knees.

Height of seat

The height of the seat should be equivalent to the distance between the posterior knee crease and the floor. Different heel heights will have a bearing on this. A seat which is too low encourages lumbar flexion whereas one that is too high prevents the user from resting his feet on the floor without pressure under the thighs (Figs. 3.40–3.42). He is then forced to sit on the front of the seat, and thereby loses the benefit of the backrest. The use of a footrest can remedy this situation, especially for people who are smaller than average. A lower chair is often preferred for relaxation purposes, but it should not be so low that getting in and out of it presents difficulties.

* Obtainable from Back Care, 151 Gwydir Street, Cambridge, CB1 2LJ. Tel: 0223-351933.

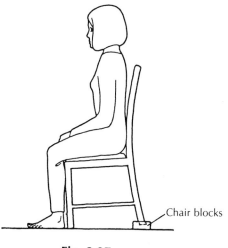

Fig. 3.37

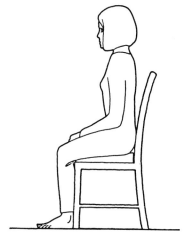

Fig. 3.38

Raising the back of the seat (by using chair blocks or a posture wedge) encourages straightening of the spine

Chair blocks

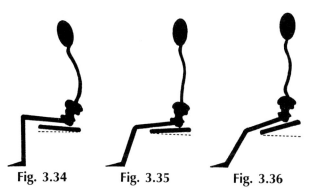

Fig. 3.34   Fig. 3.35   Fig. 3.36

A backward-sloping seat encourages the spine to bend

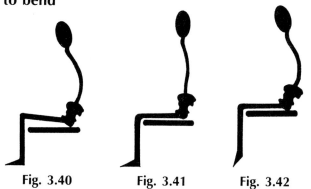

Fig. 3.40   Fig. 3.41   Fig. 3.42

A seat which is either too low or too high encourages the spine to bend

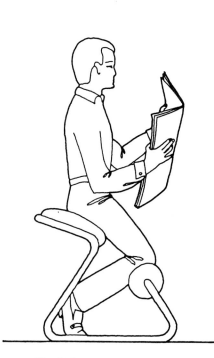

Fig. 3.39   The kneeling stool reduces intradiscal pressure.

Space under seat

There should be adequate space under the seat so that the sitter can vary the angle of knee flexion. Seats which do not allow for this, e.g. in trains or in industrial situations due to the demands of machinery, encourage a flexed posture, especially in people who have short hamstrings. With increasing knee extension, the pelvis is tilted backwards and the lumbar spine is flexed.

Depth of seat

The ideal depth of a seat is that which is the same as the measurement from the back of the knee crease to the buttocks. It is important that the user is able to sit well back into the seat as this stabilizes the back of the ischial tuberosities and sacrum, preventing the pelvis tilting too far backwards. Problems arise particularly with resting chairs when the depth is too great. In order to make contact with the backrest, the user has to flex his lumbar spine.

A seat with insufficient depth can also cause problems by giving inadequate support under the thighs, concentrating the pressure somewhere in the middle. A 'waterfall' front edge will reduce this to some extent (*see* Fig. 3.44).

Armrests

Armrests can be useful for some patients in a working situation, provided they do not interfere with the task being performed, and are essential for relaxation. When the arms are unsupported, eventually they tend to pull the upper trunk forward, increasing the load on trapezius. The sitter seeks stability by resting his forearms on his thighs for instance (Fig. 3.43).

Proper arm support (Fig. 3.44) encourages spinal extension so that greater support is obtained from the backrest of the chair and intradiscal pressure is reduced. The load on trapezius is also significantly decreased. Certainly armrests facilitate rising from sitting, which incurs a rise in intradiscal pressure, and reduce knee strain.

If the sitter is working at a table, it is essential that the armrests are low enough to go under the table. The height of the armrest should be such that it provides comfortable support to the soft muscle part of the forearms, not the elbows, without elevation of the shoulders. To facilitate rising, the armrests should extend beyond the front edge of the seat.

Height of desk

Desks tend to be less adjustable than chairs, and the office worker may find that, having suitably adjusted his chair, the height of the desk may be unacceptable. As a guide, for writing purposes, the top of the desk should be approximately 50 mm higher than the height of the elbow. Where it is important to minimize trunk flexion, a writing slope* (*see* p. 141) is invaluable. For typing purposes, the typist should be able to hold his elbows flexed between 80–90° depending on comfort, so that the fingers when on the keyboard are either level with or slightly higher than his elbows.

*Address of supplier on p. 80.

Armrests

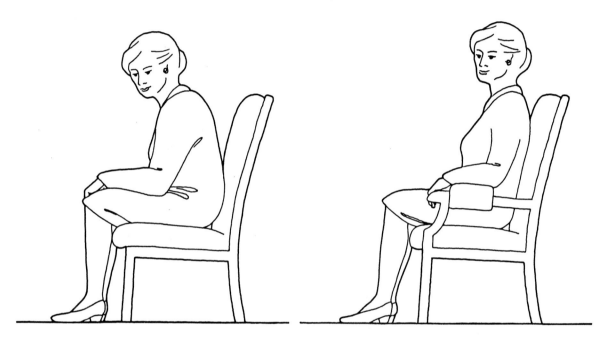

Fig. 3.43 Weight of arms pulls trunk forwards.

Fig. 3.44 Arm support encourages straighter back. Use can now be made of the back support.

Visual display units (VDUs)

The increasing use of visual display units has led to a corresponding increase in spinal problems, largely of a postural nature, particularly in the cervical and cervicothoracic regions. People are under extra risk of strain if excessive demands are placed on them, either by themselves or by others, and/or if their tolerance to physical stress is reduced because of personal or work-related factors.

When considering prevention of VDU-related musculoskeletal disorders, many factors need to be taken into account, including:

- the furniture and equipment available;
- the posture of the user;
- the amount of static muscle work involved;
- the amount of ligamentous/connective tissue strain involved;
- the numbers of hours spent using the VDU;
- the number of rest pauses taken;
- individual factors such as age, gender, personality, existing state of musculoskeletal system.

Problems have arisen with equipment mainly because of maladjustment of screens and keyboards. Units where screen and keyboard are connected close to each other in one unit create problems in that, if the keyboard is in the correct position in relation to shoulder, arm and hand position (the keyboard should be approximately at elbow height), the screen is then too low, and the user has to adopt a forward head posture (*see* pp. 52–9) in order to read the screen. The line of sight preferred by VDU users is between the horizontal and 15° downward (Grandjean *et al.*, 1983); raising the unit to accommodate this places the keyboard in too high a position, causing elevation and abduction of the shoulders (raising the muscle work of trapezius) and compensatory ulnar deviation at the wrist (Pheasant, 1991) in order for the fingers to strike the keys, causing stress over the extensor tendons and sheaths. Independent adjustments of keyboard and screen are, therefore, essential.

Another source of stress is reading from documents on one side of the desk, incurring a combination of rotation in the cervical spine and flexion in the cervical and upper thoracic spines. Loading on the neck muscles can be reduced by about one-third by using a reading stand (Fig. 3.45) (Life and Pheasant, 1984).

The posture illustrated in Fig. 3.45 incurs relatively low static muscular loads: note the slight backward inclination of the thoracolumbar spine (no more than 10–15°), which makes good use of the relatively high backrest. This posture is preferred by many VDU users.

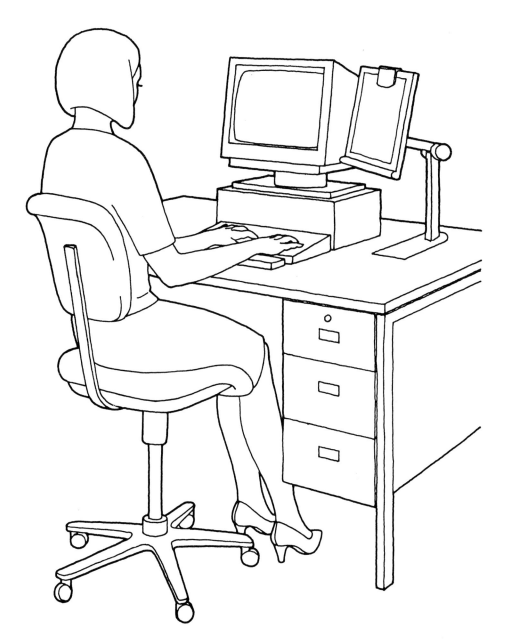

Fig. 3.45   Correct posture at VDU. Note use of reading stand to prevent neck strain.

Lower muscular activity in the upper fibres of trapezius has been demonstrated when there is slight flexion at the cervicothoracic junction and a vertical cervical spine, than with a completely upright posture (Schuldt *et al.*, 1986). The use of wrist supports also reduces muscle activity in trapezius. It is, however, important that the user experiments to see which position is most comfortable for him. Some patients prefer a more pronounced lumbar support than others, or to be more upright with a steeper seat slope. Frequent changes of position are often beneficial.

Chairs which provide adjustments to seat height and slope as well as backrest inclination are essential for keyboard users, who should receive instructions on how to adjust the chairs and on correct posture.

To offset the effects of static muscle activity or ligamentous/connective tissue strain, regular pauses from this posture are necessary, during which time the keyboard user should perform full-range movements of the head and spine so that the muscles are alternately stretched and worked dynamically to increase the circulation and to prevent the accumulation of metabolites. The exercises should be designed to suit the particular needs of each individual, e.g. some may need to include wrist and arm stretches. Suggestions to reduce spinal stress are shown in Figs. 3.46–3.51, but varying the exercises periodically is useful to prevent boredom.

The number of times the exercises need to be performed is variable. They should be used to prevent the onset of muscular fatigue, rather than just to relieve it once it has occurred. Towards the end of a working day and week, more frequent pauses are usually needed. Ideally, the individual should be helped to discover his own needs regarding the frequency and duration of the exercises. However, workers are often reluctant to take these breaks to perform exercises as they dislike being conspicuous. It is undoubtedly easier if a group of workers are all engaged in performing them, and more enjoyable to do them to music, as in Scandinavia.

For an account of current regulations which implement an E.C. directive on display screen equipment, *see* under 'Further Reading'. Negotiations between unions and management are often necessary to decide on the length and frequency of rest pauses.

In addition to, but linked with physical stress, there is a high incidence of mental stress amongst VDU users, especially when high keying rates are demanded. Sympathetic planning of work programmes which takes into consideration the need to reduce highly repetitive work, allowing variations in movements, would go a long way in preventing both musculoskeletal and mental stress.

Exercises for VDU operators

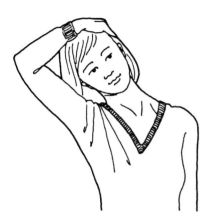

Fig. 3.46 Stretch side of neck.

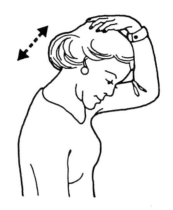

Fig. 3.48 Stretch top of neck.

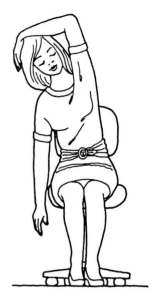

Fig. 3.50 Stretch side of trunk.

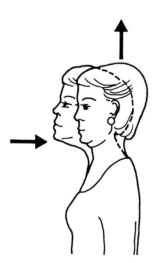

Fig. 3.47 Tuck in chin and lengthen back of neck.

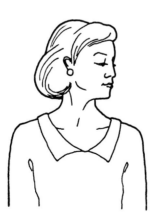

Fig. 3.49 Turn head from side to side.

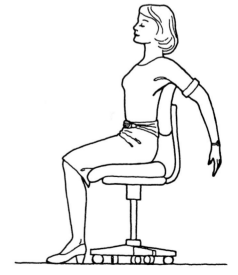

Fig. 3.51 Stretch backwards over edge of backrest.

Re-educating the sitting posture

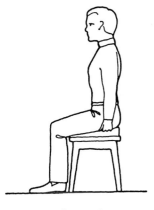

Fig. 3.52

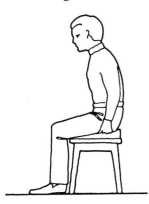

Fig. 3.53

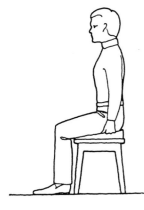

Fig. 3.54

Several teaching sessions may be necessary before the patient learns to sit in a comfortable, balanced posture, and only with diligent practice and perseverance do some patients achieve this.

The following is a method which I have found yields good results.

The patient is asked to sit on his hands with the palms uppermost so that he can feel his ischial tuberosities ('sitting bones') (Fig. 3.52). Next, he is asked to slouch and notice what happens to his 'sitting bones' (they move forwards, Fig. 3.53), then to over-arch his low back (his 'sitting bones' move backwards, Fig. 3.54). He is asked to stop when he feels the bones directly on the palms of his hands. This usually places the lumbar spine in a neutral, optimum position. Then the patient is asked to feel the weight of his trunk going *down* through these bones. Some patients' backs will collapse at this point, and it helps for the therapist to place a firm supportive hand over the patient's sacrum (Fig. 3.55), and release the support only when she finds it is not needed. Weight should also be borne by the feet.

The patient is then asked to *relax* his shoulders down and backwards—*not* to brace them backwards. To assist, the therapist can guide the movements of the scapula by placing one hand on the shoulder and the other under the inferior angle of the scapula, giving gentle resistance to it tracking downwards and medially (Fig. 3.56). For thoracic extension, the therapist places one hand over the sternum and one over the mid-thoracic spine, gently raising the chest anteriorly (Fig. 3.57). Notice the change in head posture already!

Finally, correction of head posture. The therapist places one hand under the chin and one hand under the occiput, guiding the head in an upward and backward direction (Fig. 3.58). The patient is asked to feel his neck lengthening. If he has a marked forward head posture, only a few degrees correction in one session is advisable. The therapist should hold this corrected position until she feels that the patient has stopped pulling his head forwards, and then gradually release her support. The patient has now 'learnt' the new posture and should practise this regime for two 10-minute sessions a day until correct posture is second nature to him.

It may be difficult to maintain a good posture when sitting at right angles and a posture wedge is useful (Fig. 3.52). The hips are in a neutral position at 45° (Keegan, 1953) and, with the pelvis tilted forward, the lumbar spine can also fall in a neutral position. Compare this to the elegant posture when horse-riding (*see* Fig. 3.59).

Should the patient need to bend forwards, e.g. to write at a desk, he should do so by bending from the hips (*see* Fig. 6.21, p. 141) and not from the spine (Fig. 6.20).

Posture correction must take into account the patient's pathology: people with ligamentous or discogenic pain may prefer to sit in more extension, while those with, for example, arthrosis, spinal stenosis or spondylolisthesis, may prefer more flexion. End of range positions, e.g. hyperextension, should be avoided except for very short periods.

Correction of sitting posture

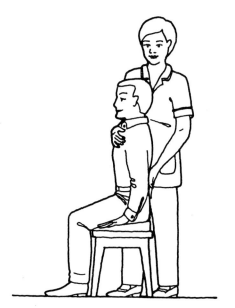

Fig. 3.55 Support low back in neutral position.

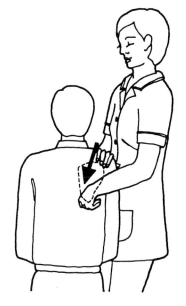

Fig. 3.56 Shoulder blade is moved downwards and inwards.

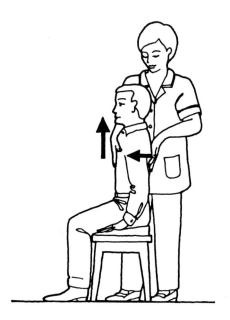

Fig. 3.57 Chest is raised.

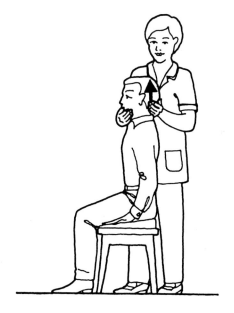

Fig. 3.58 Head is lifted upwards and backwards.

Driving

The incidence of severe back pain is twice as high in people who drive to and from work than in those who do not (Kelsey and Hardy, 1975), and in occupations such as tractor driving there is a particularly high incidence of early degenerative changes (Rosegger and Rosegger, 1960) induced by vibration. Prolonged sitting incurs higher intradiscal pressure (Fig. 2.26, p. 31), which can be further increased by poor seat design and posture. For some people, driving can be stressful, and this is then reflected in the driver's posture (Fig. 3.60).

Comfort both during driving *and* afterwards is more likely to be achieved if the backrest, lumbar support and seat angle are adjustable. However, simple alterations to existing seats can often be made which have a marked effect on comfort, especially if combined with advice on a relaxed driving posture (Fig. 3.61):

- *Seat angle*. A backward-sloping seat encourages lumbar flexion (Fig. 3.34). If this is undesirable, the angle can be altered by using a posture wedge* (2″ or 2½″ high, Fig. 3.61). Too high a wedge is undesirable as it restricts headroom.
- *Lumbar support*. These are available in different shapes and sizes.* The correct depth of support and its position either in the lumbar or sacral region depend entirely on what the patient finds comfortable. Usually, the more acute the back, the more support is needed.
- *Backrest angle*. Although some people prefer to have the backrest vertical, this is not always the case. An angle greater than 90° (*see* Fig. 3.61) which gives a lower level of intradiscal pressure is often preferred, but the patient should be instructed to rest back against the backrest, provided the visual demands are met. Varying the backrest angle on long journeys helps some patients.
- *Pedals*. In some cars, the pedals are offset to one side, causing torsion in the spine. This is something the patient should watch out for if purchasing another vehicle.
- *Depression of the clutch pedal* raises intradiscal pressure, partly due to stretching of the hamstrings which tilt the pelvis backwards and flex the lumbar spine. Moving the seat forwards lessens the hamstring stretch behind the knee, but increases it over the hip because of increased flexion. A wedge (*see* above), by decreasing hip flexion, reduces the stretch.
- *Automatic transmission* is often preferred by patients with chronic, left-sided disc problems. However, right-sided sciatica may be aggravated by automatic transmission due to adduction of the right leg, stretching the sciatic nerve.
- *Lateral tilting of the seat* causing the lumbar spine to be held in lateral flexion can be remedied by levelling the seat with a foam wedge (Fig. 3.62).
- *The headrest* should be positioned so that it is level with the eyes (Fig. 3.61) for safety: they are often too low.
- *Postural fixation*. On long journeys, a routine of getting out of the car every hour and walking around helps to prevent cumulative damage. The spine is vulnerable after long car journeys, when heavy lifting should be avoided.

* Obtainable from Back Care, 151 Gwydir Street, Cambridge CB1 2LJ. Tel: 0223-351933.

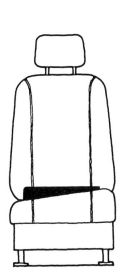

Fig. 3.62   Use of wedge
to level seat.

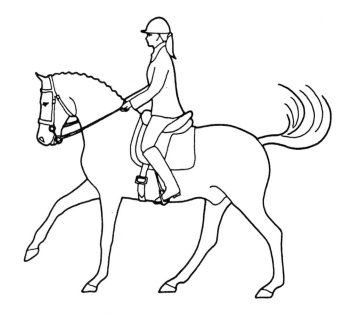

Fig. 3.59   Knees well below the hip level encourages
this balanced, elegant posture.

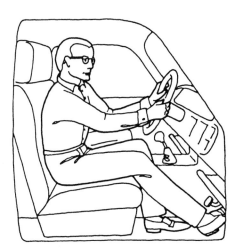

Fig. 3.60   Tense driving posture.

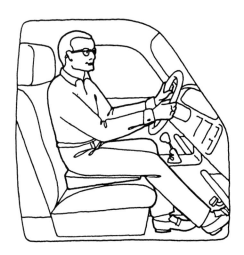

Fig. 3.61   Relaxed driving posture.

Standing

We often hear it said that the human spine has not yet become perfectly adapted to the upright posture. It is, however, more accurate to say that evolution of the human spine has not reached the stage when it can withstand the unreasonable demands imposed on it by modern technology and lifestyles.

The 'idealized' standing posture

Were all spines the same anatomically, the line of gravity would fall in the midline between the following points (Fig. 3.63) (Basmajian, 1978).

- the mastoid process;
- a point just in front of the shoulder joints;
- a point just behind the centre of the hip joints;
- a point just in front of the centre of the knee joints;
- a point just in front of the ankle joints.

Once man is actually in this idealized standing posture, little muscular activity is required to maintain it, and there is no undue stress on the ligaments.

Structure governs function, and every individual is born with his own unique structure. The lifestyle imposed on this structure is capable of changing it. If a person spends most of the day in the sitting position, eventually his joints and soft tissues will adapt to the particular posture he adopts. For example, the iliopsoas muscles, which are important in stabilizing the lumbar spine in the sitting posture, will become over-active and shorten. This, in turn, will influence the person's lesser-used standing posture; the tight iliopsoas muscles will pull the pelvis forwards, creating a state of imbalance in both muscles and joints. Also, bone remodels to some extent according to usage, and good 'use' in the way of posture is essential for a healthy spine.

The effects on the spine of the standing posture

Angle of pelvic inclination/sacral angle

The 'set' of the pelvis at the hip joints determines the angle of pelvic inclination which, in turn, determines the degree of inclination to the horizontal of the upper surface of the sacrum—called the sacral angle. On average, the size of this angle is 50–53° in the standing position (Fig. 3.64) (Hellems and Keates, 1971), but it varies considerably in different individuals and this is of paramount significance for several reasons. A larger angle means that the shearing strain of the superimposed body weight at the lumbosacral segment is greater than with smaller angles, e.g. a 35° angle means that there is the pressure to slide forward of 0.57% of the superimposed weight, whereas a 75° angle increases the strain to 0.97% (Von Lackum, 1924). The size of the sacral angle is also related to the degree of lumbar convexity. In order for the spine to assume the erect posture with an increased sacral angle, a compensatory increase in the lumbar curve has to occur (Fig. 3.65), and the centre of gravity is shifted forwards. A smaller angle results in a flattening of the lumbar curve (Fig. 3.66). Women generally have a significantly greater lordotic angle than men (Fernand and Fox, 1985).

Standing posture

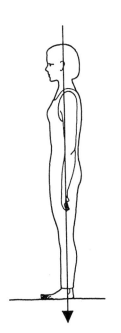

Fig. 3.63 Line of gravity in erect posture.

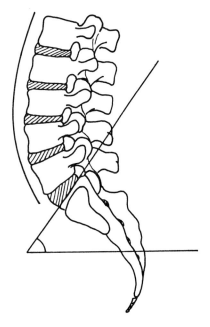

Fig. 3.64 Normal sacral angle.

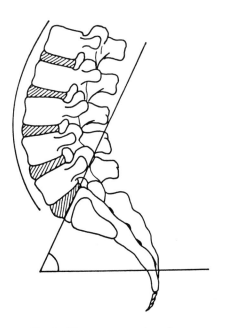

Fig. 3.65 Large sacral angle → increased lordosis.

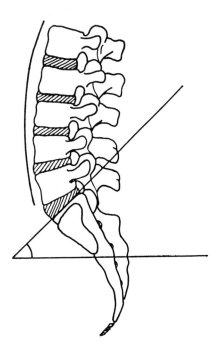

Fig. 3.66 Small sacral angle → flat back.

Muscle activity

Very little muscle activity is required to maintain the symmetrical standing posture. There is slight constant or intermittent activity in one set of trunk muscles, most frequently in the low thoracic extensors, but in 20–25% of cases in the abdominal muscles (Floyd and Silver, 1951).

The apophyseal joints

These bear a small proportion of the intervertebral compressive force in the standing posture. However, long periods of standing cause the facet tips to make contact with the laminae of the subjacent vertebra and bear about one-sixth of the compressive force (Adams and Hutton, 1980). This amount increases with more extension and when there is disc degeneration with loss of disc height. In the latter instance, as much as 70% of the intervertebral compressive force may be transmitted across the apophyseal joints (Adams and Hutton, 1983).

Ligaments

The anterior longitudinal ligament plays an important role in stabilizing the lumbar spine in the standing posture. Prolonged standing, which tends to accentuate the lumbar lordosis, places more strain on this ligament.

Intradiscal pressure

This is lower than in sitting (Fig. 2.25 on p. 31) because relatively low levels of muscle activity are involved and, as previously stated, the lumbar spine is in more extension with some of the load borne by impingement of the inferior articular facets of the apophyseal joints on the subjacent laminae.

Different skeletal types

Variations in the sacral angle have an influence on some of the following commonly observed postures:

1. *Hollow back* (Fig. 3.67). There is an increase in the sacral angle with exaggerated lumbar and thoracic curvatures.
2. *Flat back* (Fig. 3.68). The opposite is the case, i.e. the sacral angle is decreased, and the lumbar and thoracic curvatures are flattened.
3. *Long, round back* (Fig. 3.69). The spine has a long, accentuated kyphosis continuing to the lumbar region, resulting in straightening of the lumbar lordosis in the upper and middle parts of the lumbar spine. Lordosis is present only in the lower region of the lumbar spine. The stomach is pushed forward and the hip joints are somewhat in extension. The whole upper trunk is inclined to some extent backwards, and the head, cervical spine and shoulders are pushed forward to retain balance. This posture can be retained with little muscular effort by leaning onto the ligaments.
4. *Upper round back* (Fig. 3.70). Kyphosis of the thoracic spine, and particularly of its upper part, is accentuated with the head, cervical spine and shoulders thrust forwards. The lumbar curve might be slightly accentuated.

Different skeletal types

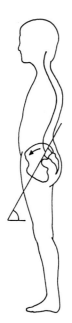

Fig. 3.67 Hollow back. Large sacral angle with exaggerated lumbar and thoracic curves.

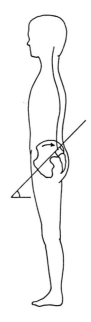

Fig. 3.68 Flat back. Small sacral angle. Lumbar and thoracic curves are flattened.

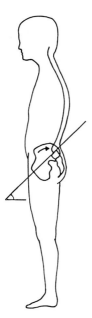

Fig. 3.69 Long, round back. Accentuated kyphosis into lumbar spine. Lordosis present in only low lumbar spine.

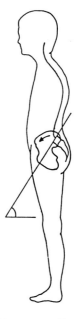

Fig. 3.70 Upper round back. Thoracic kyphosis is accentuated.

Why do people stand the way they do?

What happens to the spine when we stand will vary according to precisely how we stand. The idealized standing posture may be seen in a few individuals if they are standing for short periods, but for longer periods, such as when waiting in a queue, people frequently resort to less than perfect, and often asymmetrical, postures. Why is this, when such economical muscle activity is required if standing in a balanced posture? Prolonged standing, as we all know, is tiring, and this is due to inadequacies of our venous and arterial circulation (Basmajian, 1978) rather than to muscle fatigue. For this reason, it is less tiring to walk than to stand. The need of the body for movement makes us change position frequently rather than assume a static position. In the standing position, the apophyseal joints are not in a neutral position, but are closer to their close-packed position than in sitting. This makes the individual tend to adopt postures that reduce the lumbar lordosis (Dolan *et al.*, 1988) to place the intervertebral joints in a more neutral position, even at the expense of increasing back muscle activity and raising intradiscal pressure.

A common postural fault is standing with the weight supported mainly on one leg, the knee of which is often locked in extension with the other leg relaxed, placed slightly forward and in front of the body (Fig. 3.71). People working with the right hand commonly use the left foot as the main support and *vice versa*, and this then becomes a habit. Asymmetrical standing has a relatively low energy expenditure, which is why it is adopted, but the cost of it is strain on the ligaments of the supporting hip and knee, and spine.

Antalgic postures

In the presence of pain and muscle spasm, the patient will either consciously or subconsciously adopt an antalgic standing posture. It is futile to attempt to correct the posture at this stage before dealing with the underlying cause.

Flexion deformity

A severe flexion deformity (Fig. 3.72) often denotes some degree of discogenic pathology. Muscle spasm, however, is not solely restricted to the erectores spinae, as this would give a deformity in extension. Spasm of psoas major, the vertebral part of which arises from the lumbar spine and discs, together with spasm in the deep intersegmental muscles are also likely to be implicated.

Sciatic list

A sciatic list (Fig. 3.73) most frequently away from the painful side, but sometimes towards it, is often described by the patient as feeling as if his hip is 'out'. It has been postulated that herniation of a disc lateral to the nerve root usually produces a sciatic list away from the side of the irritated nerve root, while herniation medial to the nerve root and in an axillary position will usually produce a sciatic list toward the side of the irritated nerve root (Figs. 3.74, 3.75). Alternatively, derangement of nuclear material in the disc may have the same effect.

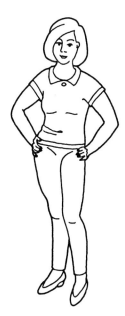

Fig. 3.71   Asymmetrical
standing.

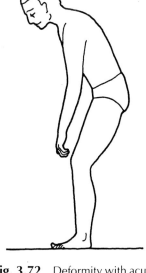

Fig. 3.72   Deformity with acute
disc pathology.

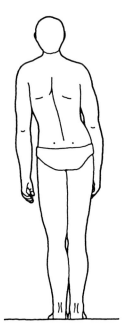

Fig. 3.73   A sciatic list.

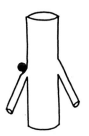

Fig. 3.74   Disc herniation lateral to nerve.
Patient relieves pain by leaning
to opposite side.

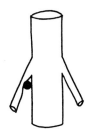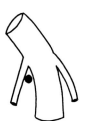

Fig. 3.75   Disc herniation in axilla of nerve
root. Patient relieves pain by
leaning to same side.

Clinically, the author has observed that in the presence of a short leg with a compensatory lumbar scoliosis, the deviation which occurs with an acute attack of back pain is such that it accentuates the deformity which was already present.

Gross sciatic lists are more likely to occur at the L4/5 segment than at the L5/S1, as the latter is stabilized by the iliolumbar ligaments. Alternating sciatic lists (i.e. varying from left to right), though relatively rare, are more frequently seen with L4/5 disc pathology. The lumbar spine is in a combination of lateral flexion with rotation.

Hip and knee bent on the painful side (Fig. 3.76)

The patient has difficulty in putting his foot to the ground, and walks on the ball of it to avoid stretching the sciatic nerve.

Combined flexion and lateral flexion deformity (Fig. 3.77)

This usually indicates lumbar disc pathology.

Effect of different height heels on standing posture

The heel height of the shoes worn by some patients can have a significant effect on pain response. It is often assumed that wearing high, as opposed to low, heels has the effect of increasing the lumbar lordosis and, although this may be so when high heels have just been put on, it has been shown in a biomechanical study that when a one-hour adaptation period in shoes with varying heel heights was allowed (Fig. 3.78), the reverse occurred to the lordotic curves in women (Bendix *et al.*, 1984). It was hypothesized that with high-heeled shoes, adaptation occurred by plantarflexion at the ankle joints, shifting the legs and trunk backwards. To compensate for this reaction, the upper trunk inclined forward, giving rise to a decrease in the lumbar curve. The above study was carried out on healthy young women with, presumably, no history of back pain. The presence of muscle spasm and the flexibility of the patient's spine may well have some bearing on how the back reacts with different heel heights. It is wiser, therefore, to simply point out to the patient that different height heels may affect the pain response, and let the patient discover which particular height is most suitable, rather than be dogmatic.

Wearing of cushioned insoles

Patients who have severe spinal pain will notice the difference between walking on a cushioned surface, such as grass, and walking on concrete paving slabs. Wearing shoes with cushioned insoles (or crêpe-soled shoes) as opposed to harder soles can simulate the softer surface. The former reduce the effect of jarring—in the neck as well as lower in the spine and lower limb joints.

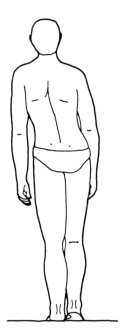

Fig. 3.76 Patient with sciatica.

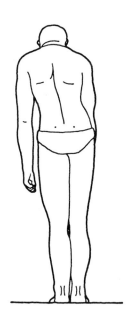

Fig. 3.77 Disc pathology: patient is bent forwards and to one side.

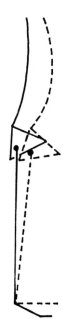

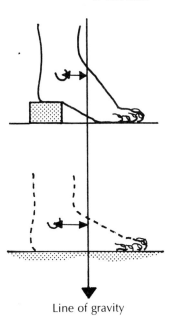

Line of gravity

Fig. 3.78 Effect of different heel heights on back. With increasing heel height, line of gravity shifts backwards → reduction in pelvic inclination → flattening of back. (Adapted from T. Bendix, S. S. Sørensen and K. Klausen, 1984. Lumbar curve, trunk muscles and line of gravity with different heel heights. *Spine,* **9**, 2, 226.)

Correction of standing posture

The most damaging postural fault is the tendency to shorten the natural curves of the spine (Fig 3.79) and, in so doing, over-compressing the anterior or posterior elements instead of maintaining a balance between them. Although aesthetically displeasing, most of the postures commonly seen (p. 95) show some evidence of this.

Once we are familiar with the structure of the patient's spine, it is unnecessary and often embarrassing for him to remain disrobed. Comfortable and unrestrictive clothing should be worn.

Before attempting posture training in standing, the patient should have mastered pelvic control in an easier position such as in crook lying. Once he can alternately flatten and then arch the low back in this position, he should then progress to flattening it into a neutral position; then, maintaining this, he should attempt to straighten first one leg, keeping the heel on the supporting surface, and then the other (Fig. 3.80). If the low back starts to arch during this procedure, the patient should stop the movement, recorrect the neutral position of the lumbar spine and then continue to straighten his leg. The patient may find it helpful to place one hand under his low back to feel the movement. The ease with which he can do this will give the therapist some idea as to his capacity to control his pelvic and lumbar movements in the standing position.

The patient should stand with his legs turned out slightly, so that the feet are approximately at 30° to each other. First, attention is directed to the weight distribution through the feet. Weight should, of course, be taken equally through both feet. Often it falls too much on the balls of the feet and the patient should be asked to transfer more weight gradually onto the heels. The therapist can guide this by supporting him round the pelvis and guiding him slowly backwards. If the knees are tightly braced back, the patient is asked to let them come forwards slightly, i.e. flex them a few degrees, still maintaining correct weight distribution through the feet.

Flexing the knees albeit slightly gives the low back the opportunity to adopt a more neutral position which lengthens the spine. Releasing the low back to allow this to happen is important, and tilting the pelvis backwards by using abdominal muscle contraction (Fig. 3.81) may help initially to give this feeling, but it is inadvisable for him to hold a static abdominal contraction for too long as this simply causes unwanted tension. The instruction, 'Let the back lengthen' is useful. To assist the patient in this movement, the therapist stands at his side, placing one hand over his sacrum and the other over his abdomen and guides the pelvic tilting. Balance is gained by correct positioning and adequate relaxation of tense muscles, e.g. erector spinae, rather than by crudely tightening muscles.

Next, the thoracic area. Similar correction follows to that in the sitting position (*see* pp. 88–9), ending with neck posture (Fig. 3.82).

Correction of standing posture

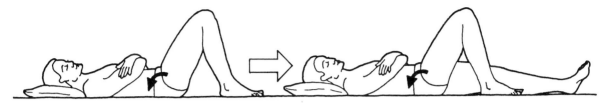

Fig. 3.80 Pelvic control. First the neutral position of the low back is found by arching and flattening it, then stopping in the mid-position. This is then held as one leg is straightened.

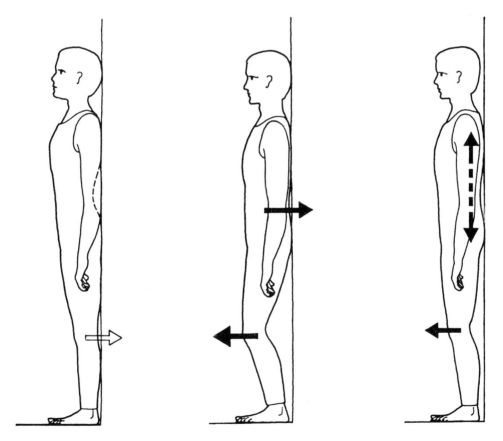

Fig. 3.79 Curves of spine are shortened: poor posture.

Fig. 3.81 Bend knees slightly and flatten low back against wall. Back of head should be stretched upwards with chin in.

Fig. 3.82 Relax, but maintain length of spine.

The patient must practise this procedure at home regularly until it becomes second nature. Standing with the back to a wall and the feet a few inches away may help in the early stages: contact with the wall gives the patient some reassurance when he is practising on his own. Having gained this, he must then rely on proprioceptive impulses from the skin and joints.

We rarely just 'stand', but this balanced standing posture forms the basis for other movements performed from the standing position. The patient should try to maintain this posture while at the same time moving his arms forwards, out to the side and behind him. Lifting the arms up above the head (as when reaching up to a high shelf) is usually accompanied by arching of the low back (Fig. 3.83), and this should be practised with the lumbar spine in a neutral position (Fig. 3.84).

It is also useful to demonstrate to the patient in front of a long mirror what happens to the spine when we carry a heavy bag in one arm (Fig. 3.85). The muscles on the opposite side of the spine have to compensate by overcontracting to maintain balance. Sharing the load evenly between two bags (Fig. 3.86) involves less muscle activity, as does carrying the load closer to the body (Fig. 3.87).

Many therapists have found posture training unsatisfactory and the results disappointing. I am sure that this is largely because insufficient time has been allowed to re-educate the patient's postural awareness. We have spent all our lives accumulating postural defects: these cannot be eradicated by a few minutes' instruction at the end of a treatment session.

We as therapists must be prepared to work *with* the patient during posture training and not rely solely on verbal instruction. In other words, we must be prepared to act as role models.

Often the patient is unaware of any increased muscle tension because overcontraction of a muscle diminishes muscle spindle activity, so that there is an absence of feedback (Barlow, 1955). Some patients have less proprioceptive awareness than others, and need more time spent on them; frequently these are the ones who eventually derive the most benefit from posture training.

Pain produced by standing

Spinal deformities in the foot are frequently one of the causative factors of spinal pain in the standing position and when walking by affecting the mechanical function of the leg, hip, pelvis and spine. For example, abnormal pronation of the subtalar joint can prevent the normal locking mechanism of the subtalar and midtarsal joints, which is necessary during the propulsive phase of walking. This results in instability of the foot, and loss of its ability to become fixed against the ground, and to help propel the body's weight efficiently. Twisting and shearing of the bones in the foot can cause rotary stresses, which are transmitted via the hips and pelvis to the lumbar spine during standing and walking. The gluteal muscles can be overstretched and weakened, causing an increase in the sacral angle and an increased lordosis. When the patient walks, his apophyseal joints in the low lumbar spine may be in their close-packed position during the hip extension phase, with resultant stress and pain. An orthosis for the affected foot may need to be prescribed to create optimum function. When the base on which the patient is standing is stable, posture correction is facilitated.

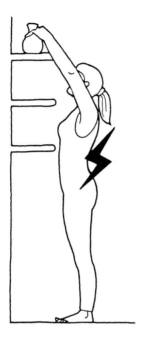

Fig. 3.83 Low back tends to arch when reaching upwards.

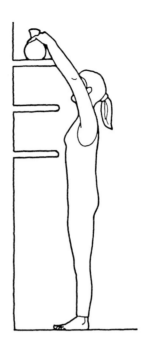

Fig. 3.84 Flatten back while reaching upwards.

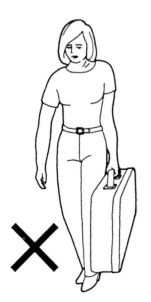

Fig. 3.85 High muscle activity needed to balance one heavy bag.

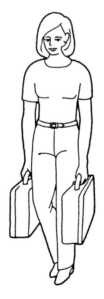

Fig. 3.86 Two lighter bags.

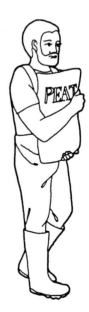

Fig. 3.87 Carry loads close to body to reduce muscle activity.

If the standing position produces the patient's low back pain, it may either be relieved by flattening the low back as shown above (e.g. in the lordosis syndrome or arthrotic back) or by tilting the pelvis forwards and deliberately arching the back (in the early discogenic syndrome). Although asymmetrical standing would never be the first choice, sometimes it is the only way that some patients can get relief from symptoms. If so, and if possible, it is better that the patient alternates the legs when standing for long periods. Body symmetry can to some extent be maintained by placing one leg a short distance forward and then rocking backwards and forwards so that the body weight falls alternately on one leg then the other (*see* Fig. 3.88).

Bending/leaning forwards

Many activities at home and work involve working over a sink or bench. It is often the slight bend (Fig. 3.89) that causes problems — erector spinae contracts to hold this position, whereas at full bend it is inactive. Inability to put the feet under the working surface increases the hazard. Ideally, working surfaces should be of such height that bending is minimized, and there should be plenty of foot room, e.g. under kitchen units. To a certain extent, the patient can compensate by standing with a wide base (which automatically lowers his body) and by tilting his pelvis backwards to reduce the shearing forces on the lumbar spine. Physiotherapists can also do this when they perform mobilizing techniques on their patients (Fig. 3.90). Placing one knee up on the plinth for support is a good way of reducing strain on the back (Fig. 3.91).

References

Adams M. A., Hutton W. C. (1980). The effect of posture on the role of the apophyseal joints in resisting intervertebral compressive force. *J. Bone Joint Surg.*, **62B**, 358.

Adams M. A., Hutton W. C. (1983). The mechanical function of the lumbar apophyseal joints. *Spine* **8**, 327.

Andersson B. J. G., Murphy R. W., Ortengren R. *et al.* (1979). The influence of backrest inclination and lumbar support on lumbar lordosis. *Spine*, **4**, 1, 52.

Barlow W. (1955). Psychosomatic problems in postural re-education. *Lancet* **ii**, 24 Sept., 659.

Basmajian J. V. (1978). *Muscles Alive: Their Functions revealed by Electromyography*, 4th edn. Baltimore: Williams & Wilkins.

Bendix T., Sorensen S. S., Klausen K. (1984). Lumbar curve, trunk muscles, and line of gravity with different heel heights. *Spine*, **9**, 2, 223.

Dolan P., Adams M. A., Hutton W. C. (1988). Commonly adopted postures and their effect on the lumbar spine. *Spine*, **13**, 2, 197.

Editorial (1979). Stay young by good posture. *New Scientist*, **82**, 544.

Fernand R., Fox D. E. (1985). Evaluation of lumbar lordosis. A prospective and retrospective study. *Spine*, **10**, 9, 799.

Floyd W. F., Silver P. H. S. (1951). Function of erectores spinae in flexion of the trunk. *Lancet*, **i**, 133.

Grandjean E., Hünting W., Piderman M. (1983). VDT workstation design: preferred settings and their effects. *Human Factors*, **25**, 161.

Hellems H. K., Keates T. E. (1971). Measurement of the normal lumbosacral angle. *Am. J. Roentgenol.*, **133**, 642.

Janda V. (1988). Muscles and cervicogenic pain syndromes. In *Physical Therapy of the Cervical and Thoracic Spine* (Grant R., ed.), Edinburgh: Churchill Livingstone.

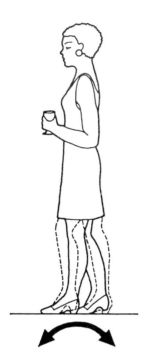

Fig. 3.88   Rock backwards and forwards on feet to relieve pain when standing.

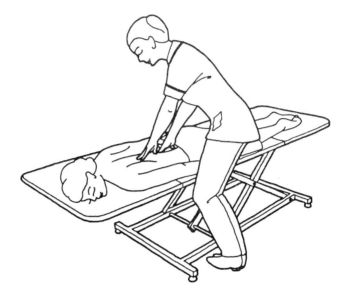

Fig. 3.90   Physiotherapists take note! Keep lumbar spine in a neutral position when performing mobilizing techniques.

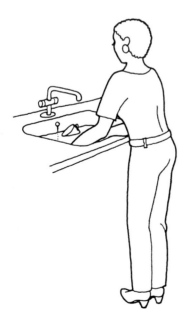

Fig. 3.89   Leaning forwards slightly incurs high muscle work in back.

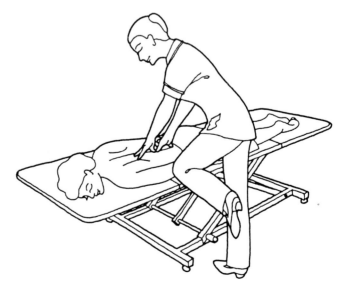

Fig. 3.91   One knee up on plinth helps to prevent back strain.

Keagy R. D., Brumlik J., Bergan J. L. (1966). Direct electromyography of the psoas major muscle in man. *J. Bone Joint Surg.*, **48-A**, 1377.

Keegan J. J. (1953). Alterations to the lumbar curve related to posture and seating. *J. Bone Joint Surg.*, **35**, 589.

Kelsey J. L., Hardy R. J. (1975). Driving of motor vehicles as a risk factor for acute herniated lumbar intervertebral disc. *Amer. J. Epidemiol.*, **102**, 63.

Life M. A., Pheasant S. T. (1984). An integrated approach to the study of posture in keyboard operation. *Applied Ergonomics*, **15**, 83.

Lundervold A. J. S. (1951). *Electromyographic Investigations of Position and Manner of Working in Typewriting.* Oslo: W. Brøggers Boktrykkeri A/S.

Nachemson A. (1965). The effect of forward leaning on lumbar intra-discal pressure. *Acta Orthop. Scand.*, **35**, 314.

Pheasant S. (1991). *Ergonomics, Work and Health,* London: Macmillan Press.

Rosegger R., Rosegger S. (1960). Health effects of tractor driving. *J. Agricult. Eng. Res.*, **5**, 241.

Schoberth H. (1962). *Sitzhaltung, Sitzschaden, Sitzmobel,* Berlin: Springer Verlag.

Schuldt K., Ekholm J., Harms-Ringdahl K. *et al.* (1986). Effects of changes in sitting work posture on static neck and shoulder muscle activity. *Ergonomics*, **29**, 12, 1525.

Von Lackum H. L. (1924). The lumbosacral region. *J. Am. Med. Ass.* **82**, 1109.

Wyke B. D. (1981). The neurology of the joints: a review of general principles. *Clin. Rheum. Dis.*, **7**, 23.

Further Reading

Health and Safety (Display Screen Equipment) Regulations (1992). HMSO.

4
Lifting

Most people think they already know the correct way to lift (although they may not do it!): 'Keep the back straight, and bend the knees'; in other words, squat. Why, then, are so many spinal injuries caused by incorrect lifting? Up to 30% of all industrial injuries occur during the manual transport of loads (Hayne, 1981).

One of the reasons is that the squat lift is infrequently used, because it requires a greater expenditure of energy than the stoop (straight knees, bent back) lift due to greater body weight being displaced vertically (Troup, 1977). People naturally try to minimize their energy expenditure. With the squat lift, fatigue is induced earlier and consequently encourages a poor lifting technique. There is, therefore, a reluctance to lift in a way which may feel unnatural. Another important consideration is that because high forces act on the knee joints during a squat lift, patients with degenerative changes in their knees often have difficulty lifting this way.

Leverage

One lifting method alone does not suit each individual. However, there is one general principle which should be applied to all lifts: **the load to be lifted should be kept as close as possible to the body**. The greater the horizontal distance of the object from the body, the greater the stress on the spine, and the greater the risk of injury (Fig. 4.1). This principle of levers can be explained to the patient by using the analogy of a crane. During spinal flexion, the L5/S1 disc acts as the main fulcrum of movement. The force exerted on it is the product of the load to be lifted, including the weight of the trunk above the disc, and its distance from the disc. The back muscles have to balance and lift the load, but they act on a short lever. Therefore, if the load to be lifted is at some distance from the body, a considerably stronger muscular force is necessary to lift it, with a proportionate increase in intradiscal pressure. This is why, for example, lifting a few dinner plates at arm's length can impose more stress on the spine than a heavier weight lifted close to the body.

Whenever possible, therefore, we should lift from between the knees, rather than in front of them (Figs. 4.2, 4.3) to reduce the lever arm of the load and the stress on the spine. This increases the strength of the lifting action and reduces the likelihood of the load getting out of control. Sometimes it is necessary to bend one of the knees in order to achieve this, e.g. lifting a child from the car or a patient up the bed (*see* Figs. 4.4, 4.5).

Sizes of containers also affect leverage (see Figs. 4.6, 4.7). A large container necessitates holding the arms well in front of the body or out to the side. In an industrial situation, container size should be kept as small as possible.

Leverage

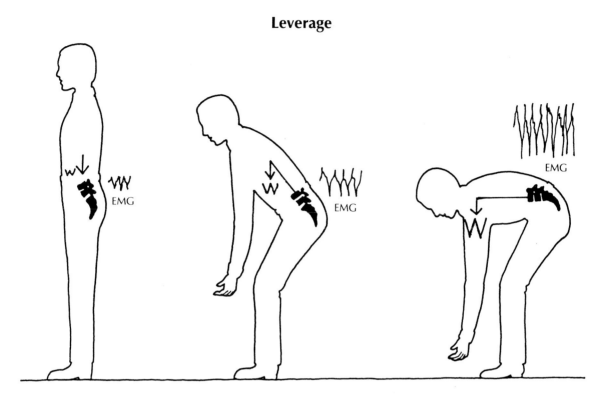

Fig. 4.1 A load requires increased back muscle activity when it is held further in front of the body.

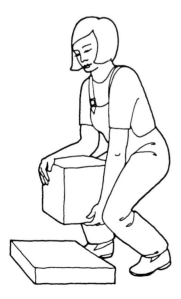

Fig. 4.2 Short lever → less stress on spine.

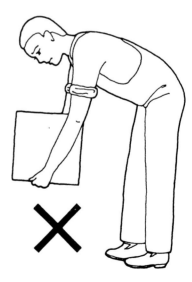

Fig. 4.3 Long lever → stress on spine.

The Individual's Capacity for Safe Lifting

Each person has a capacity for safe lifting which is unique to him, and it is important that the therapist explores with him what his maximum safe capacity is. An individual's capacity to lift safely depends on the following factors.

Gender

Women are approximately 30% weaker than men of equivalent height, weight and training (Hayne, 1981). Guidelines have been laid down recommending maximum weights and work loads for industrial workers: unfortunately, no such data have been compiled for housewives/mothers!

Body types

The slender, weaker muscled type of person is more at risk from lifting accidents than the stockier type with strong muscles, because of the longer leverages involved and poorer muscle tone.

Age

With ageing, the spine loses some of its shock absorbing properties, mainly due to a reduction in water content, relative increase in collagen in the discs, and a decrease in bone strength, especially in women. The ability to lift heavy loads safely is thereby lessened. It is not always easy to convey this to older patients, who may have been very active in the past and are eager to continue with DIY work. It is useful to point out to these patients that their quality of life will, in fact, be enhanced by being realistic about their capacities rather than by incurring unnecessary debility.

Pathological condition of the spine

Certain pathological conditions, in particular where the intervertebral discs are involved, will influence the person's lifting ability. Repetitive heavy lifting during the adolescent years (e.g. farm labouring) is likely to be one of the causes of Schmorl's nodes or intravertebral disc prolapses, (Fig. 4.8; see p. 42).

In older spines, the nuclei in discs that show signs of degeneration may be unable to behave hydrostatically under compressive loading. This places a larger tensile stress on the outer annular fibres which then show increased bulging, since they lose more height than normal discs (Köller et al., 1981). Subsequent narrowing of the disc space increases pressure between the facets of the apophyseal joints (Fig. 4.9), which may then be a source of pain. Increased annular bulging may be sufficient to compromise the spinal nerve root in its intervertebral foramen, causing referred pain. Patients who have undergone surgery for excision of the disc or chemonucleolysis with subsequent disc space narrowing are also prone to this increase in stress across the apophyseal joints.

Pathological changes in the spine are often similar to those which occur with normal ageing, and their presence does not necessarily mean that the patient should never lift, but rather that he should respect the spine's limitations. During an acute attack, lifting, with a consequent rise in intradiscal pressure, slows down the natural healing process, and can convert an annular prolapse into a nuclear extrusion (see pp. 28–9). The turnover of collagen in the disc is very slow, and recurrent bouts of back pain in patients with discogenic pathology are largely due to overstressing the disc during its slow healing process.

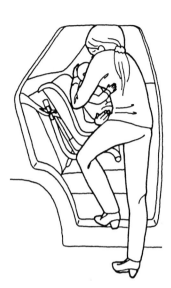

Fig. 4.4   Get close to child –
lift one foot up.

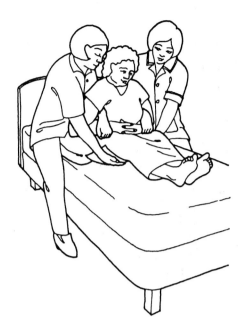

Fig. 4.5   The through-arm
lift.

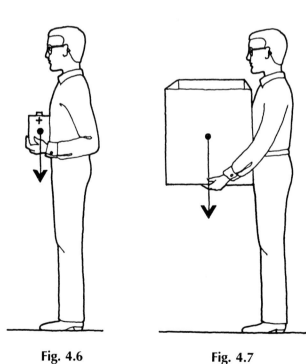

Fig. 4.6   **Fig. 4.7**

Sizes of containers affect leverage. Small containers (Fig. 4.6)
can be held with their centre of gravity close to the body.

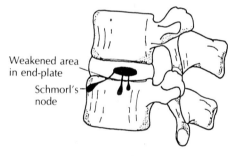

Weakened area
in end-plate

Schmorl's
node

Fig. 4.8

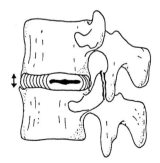

Fig. 4.9   Narrowing of disc space increases
pressure on facet joints.

The precondition of the spine

In the main, trauma to the spine is not caused by one single episode. The patient may believe that simply bending to pick up his shaving brush caused his back to 'go', but this was undoubtedly the last straw in a series of repetitive minor traumata.

The spine has the capacity to 'store up' trauma without registering pain. Annular distortion (Figs. 4.10, 4.11) and some loss of disc height occur following repetitive movements, such as those involved in lifting, and the time taken for the disc to regain its 'normal' state depends on how the patient uses his back afterwards, and the magnitude and duration of loads then applied to it, including the postures taken up. If he rests supine afterwards, the disc has a chance to reinflate.

It is possible, however, that even a night's sleep does not completely restore some discs, which are then more vulnerable to injury the next day. Indeed, patients often report that their backs 'went' a day or two *after* heavy lifting. There is a peak incidence of back injuries between 9.00–11.00 am (Evans and Pearcy, 1978) when the disc's fluid content is abnormally high and, therefore, more resistant to bending stresses (Andersson and Schultz, 1979). In the early morning, therefore, spinal flexion stresses may be less safe than later in the day.

Symptoms such as discomfort, aching, or a feeling of tiredness in the back often precede more serious back injuries, and the patient would be well advised to be alert to these warning signals and take rests in supine or crook lying.

Training

People who are most likely to sustain back injuries are the unprepared, unskilled, young people and those in their first year or so of a new job (Blow and Jackson, 1971; Magora, 1974). Patterns of movement are laid down very early in life, and physical education in schools could play an important role in encouraging smooth, well-coordinated movements. In an industrial situation, training in good lifting techniques is essential, but these should be regularly monitored to ensure that proper methods become a habit.

General Guidelines for Lifting

Before any lift is attempted, the patient should consider the following factors to make sure it is safely executed.

Do I need help? (Fig. 4.12)

Bearing in mind that lifting accounts for up to 30% of all industrial accidents, and that lifting in the home probably accounts for far more, we should stop for a moment to consider the lift, especially with heavy loads:

- Is the load within my safe capacity? (*see* p. 110)
- If not—can another person assist me?
    —is there a hoist or other mechanical device that could be used?

The position of the load (Figs. 4.13, 4.14)

It is impossible for most people to lift loads from floor level without some flexion occurring in the lumbar spine, even when the squat lift is used, and the initial phase of such a lift is risky. Where repetitive lifting is necessary, loads should be placed at or above knee height.

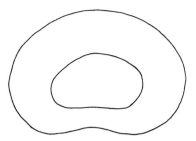

Fig. 4.10   Cross-section of normal disc.

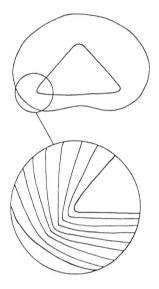

Fig. 4.11   Distortion of disc after bending or lifting.

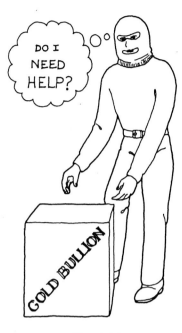

Fig. 4.12

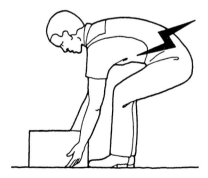

Fig. 4.13   Lifting from floor level always involves bending back, even when the knees are bent.

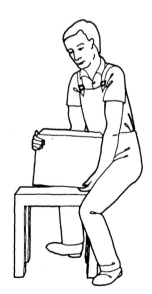

Fig. 4.14   Loads at or above knee height are safer to lift.

Plan the lift

Suitable clothing should be worn (Fig. 4.2, p. 109) that is loose enough to allow free movement but tight enough to avoid catching. Loose belts or loose sleeves can be hazardous. If the object to be lifted is dirty, e.g. when gardening, the tendency is to hold it at a distance from the body to avoid soiling clean clothes. Nurses' uniforms, for example, should permit them sufficient freedom of movement to use a wide base and get one knee up if necessary. Gloves may be necessary to protect the hands from sharp objects; they should fit properly to assist a firm grip. Attention must also be given to footwear: appropriate shoes that encourage a firm, balanced stance are necessary. Jerky movements caused by stumbling when wearing too high-heeled shoes (Fig. 4.15) or flip-flops can cause damage. In an industrial situation, shoes or boots with non-slip soles and safety toe caps may be needed.

Working area

The workplace should be uncluttered to avoid the worker having to reach out to lift a load or tripping over objects on the floor (Fig. 4.16).

Get close to the load
(Fig. 4.17)

This is by far the most important point to remember for correct lifting (*see* Leverage on p. 108). Whether or not the knees are bent or straight makes little difference to intradiscal pressure (Andersson *et al.*, 1977; Nachemson, 1976), but lifting with the arms outstretched as opposed to close to the body demands stronger contraction of erector spinae and, therefore, raises intradiscal pressure considerably. This also applies when putting down the load as well as lifting it.

Stand with a stable base
(Fig. 4.18)

Stability is essential to enable the lift to be carried out smoothly. The feet should be apart, with the load in-between the knees if possible to keep it close to the body.

Good grip (Fig. 4.19)

The design of containers should be in sympathy with the person having to lift them. Handles and grips placed in strategic positions can increase the grip strength of the lifter. Where a good grip is not readily available, the object should be tilted onto its side to obtain a firm grip on the opposite side. The texture of the surface is also important, rough textures being easier to grip than smooth ones. To increase grip strength, the lifter should use the palms of his hands together with fingers and thumbs.

The position of the feet

The lifter should, if possible, stand so that he is facing the direction in which he needs to carry the load, with one foot behind the load and the other to the side of it, the forward foot facing the direction of travel (Fig. 4.19). If he then has to move the load to the side, he should do so by turning his feet and not his torso. Twisting or laterally flexing when lifting, carrying or lowering the load further increases intradiscal pressure and is often the 'final straw' which causes a disc to herniate.

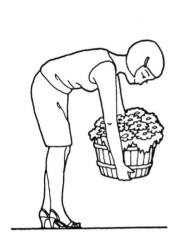

Fig. 4.15   Wear suitable clothes!

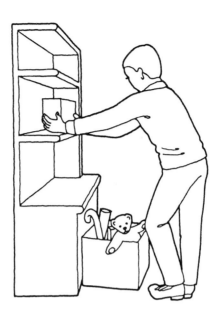

Fig. 4.16   Cluttered areas necessitate reaching out to lift objects.

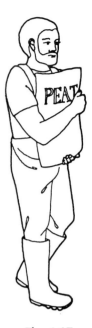

Fig. 4.17
GET CLOSE TO THE LOAD.

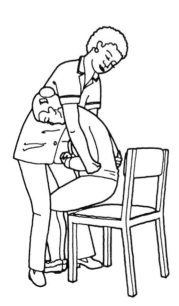

Fig. 4.18   Stand with a stable base.

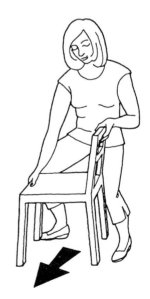

Fig. 4.19   Stand facing direction of travel. Get a good grip.

The lift itself

The lift should be carried out at a natural speed using an integrated movement combining some hip and knee flexion with the lumbar spine usually in a neutral position and with the chin in. This will vary somewhat according to the particular lift and the individual. If the above factors have been adhered to, the lifter will assume a posture, individual to his own body structure, which will be right and efficient for him. The lumbar spine is usually best in a neutral position. Consciously bracing the abdominal muscles to raise intra-abdominal pressure and thereby reduce intradiscal pressure (Bartelink, 1957) may help to stabilize the spine in some individuals (Fig. 4.20). Some selected patients need to have their lumbar spines in more extension when lifting, but lifting heavy loads in extension should be avoided, as it causes excessive pressure on the apophyseal joints. It will be observed that weight lifters use a belt to *prevent* hyperextension.

Patients often believe that they should always keep their backs vertical during a lift. This is a fallacy and, if adhered to, could mean that the load is kept at a distance from the body. They should be shown how to move with a load so that it feels part of them.

Is the patient fit to lift?

Patients should only return to work involving lifting when they have:

- *Paravertebral and abdominal* muscles which are strong enough for their particular tasks ahead of them. The need for strength anteriorly and laterally in the spine may come as a surprise to some patients, and the role of the abdominal muscles in bracing and providing nature's own corset needs emphasis. The use of a temporary orthopaedic corset may be indicated for some patients who have had recurrent bouts of severe back pain.
- Strong *glutei and quadriceps* muscles to enable them to execute the lift.

Correct lifting has to be taught by the therapist doing it with the patient, not simply by telling him, however lucidly, what to do. The patient then has to practise the correct movement repeatedly until it becomes second nature to him. Practising the movement using a very light weight is by far the best way of strengthening the glutei and quadriceps muscles, as they are then working in that functional capacity. Another useful method for patients with arthritic knees is gentle squatting in a painfree range in a swimming pool, using the assistance of buoyancy (Fig. 4.21).

References

Andersson G. B. J., Ortengren R., Nachemson A. (1977). Intradiscal pressure, intra-abdominal pressure and myoelectric back muscle activity related to posture and loading. *Clin. Orthop.*, **129**, 156.

Andersson G. B., Schultz A. B. (1979). Effects of fluid injection on mechanical properties of intervertebral discs. *J. Biomech.*, **12**, 453.

Bartelink J. V. (1957). The role of abdominal pressure in relieving the pressure on the lumbar intervertebral discs. *J. Bone Jt. Surg.*, **39-B**, 4, 718.

Blow R. J., Jackson J. M. (1971). An analysis of back injuries in registered dock workers. *Proc. Roy. Soc. Med.*, **64**, 735.

Evans J., Pearcy M. (1978). The back problem and other musculo-skeletal injuries at Mount Isa Mines Limited. Department of Bioengineering, University of Strathclyde, Glasgow, Scotland (unpublished report).

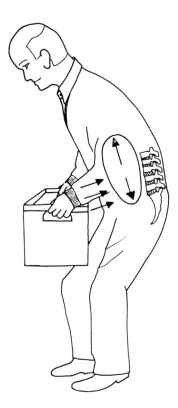

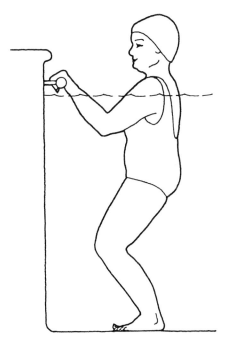

Fig. 4.20   Brace abdominal muscles
to raise intra-abdominal
pressure.

Fig. 4.21   Semi-squats in a swimming
pool strengthen knees
without strain.

Hayne C. R. (1981). Manual transport of loads by women. *Physiotherapy*, **67**, 8, 226.

Köller W., Funke F., Hartmann F. (1981). Das verformungsverhalten vom lumbalen menschlichen Zwischenwirbelscheiben unter langein-wirkender axialer dynamischer Druckkraft. *Z. Orthop.*, **119**, 206.

Magora A. (1974). Investigation of the relation between low back pain and occupation, 6. Medical history and symptoms. *Scand. J. Rehab. Med.*, **6**, 81.

Nachemson A. L. (1976). The lumbar spine. An orthopaedic challenge. *Spine* 1, **59**.

Troup J. D. G. (1977). Dynamic factors in the analysis of stoop and crouch lifting methods: a methodological approach to the development of safe materials handling standards. *Orthop. Clin. N. Am.*, **8**, 201.

5
Exercises

By definition, an exercise is a 'course of movements for the sake of strength or health'. The numerous movements we perform during the day, often repetitively, are not considered to be 'exercises' because they are not performed for reasons of strength or health. It is these same movements, however, which are collectively responsible for whatever state of imbalance in muscle strength and joint range occurs throughout the musculoskeletal system. If we repetitively perform any series of movements, we will strengthen and often over-use the muscle groups that are responsible. Everyday movements should not, therefore, be seen in isolation from exercises.

When a patient is asked to carry out an exercise, he should realize that the intention is for it to have a beneficial effect on his movements during the rest of the day, not just while he is doing the exercise. For example, if a patient presents with pain brought on by flexion and eased by extension exercises (Figs. 5.1–5.4), he should learn to offset any damage caused by repetitive flexion movements during the day by extending his spine. Being taught the exercises without the follow-through use during everyday activities is of little value, and is one of the main reasons why some exercise regimes fail.

Not all patients will be enthusiastic about doing exercises, and the personality of the patient should be respected. Compliance is greater if the patient is given just one or two exercises to do which are simple to perform. Lists of indiscriminate exercises are enough to put anyone off. It should also be borne in mind that if the patient is working in, say, an office, he may not wish to lie down in front of his colleagues to perform exercises, although doing one or two standing up may be acceptable. In some cases, however, it is probably better for the therapist to concentrate on some other aspect of back care, e.g. ergonomics! Exercises that are performed with an ill-will often have a detrimental effect.

Not every patient with back pain should be given spinal exercises as a matter of course. Especially in the acute stage, some exercises may even cause a bulging disc to herniate. The therapist should consider her reason for prescribing exercises, and find out if the patient is already doing his 'daily dozen'. It is not within the scope of this guide to name the numerous exercises that may help spinal conditions, but those illustrated are the basic and essential ones.

A simple, written account of the exercise (Fig. 5.5) should be given to the patient after he has been taught the exercise:

ABDOMINAL BRACING

Starting position: Lie on back on firm surface, with knees bent.
Exercise: Brace your tummy muscles so that your back flattens against the surface. Hold for 10 seconds—keep breathing!—then relax.
Caution: If back or leg pain is increased—STOP doing this exercise.
No. of repetitions: _____ Times per day: _____

Fig. 5.5

Pain-relief using extension postures and exercises

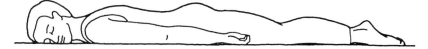

Fig. 5.1 Prone-lying.

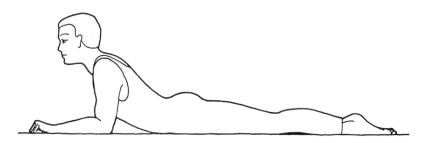

Fig. 5.2 Prone-lying with upper trunk raised.

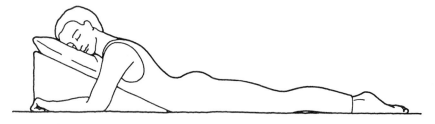

Fig. 5.3 Elbow-support prone-lying.

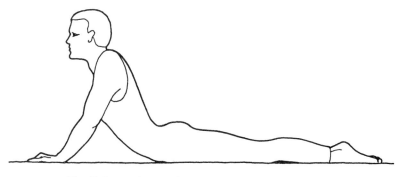

Fig. 5.4 Push up with arms into passive extension of the lumbar spine.

General Principles

- Exercises should be performed smoothly and rhythmically.
- Exercises involving flexion *and* extension should not be given together in one session until the effect of one movement has been assessed, except when exercises are given for generalized stiffness.
- The effect of each exercise should be assessed at a follow-up appointment.

Exercises for Pain Relief

The most frequently used pain-relieving exercises and positions (*see* pp. 67–9) involve either flexion or extension of the thoracolumbar spine.

Pain relief using extension

The series of positions and exercises shown in Figs. 5.1–5.4, 5.6 and 5.7 are often effective for the patient whose back pain is increased by repetitive spinal flexion and eased by extension in a selected position, e.g. with early discogenic problems.

The choice of starting position is critical in some cases. If the pain is severe, or if a flexion deformity is present, extension in standing may exacerbate the pain, whereas it may be relieved by prone-lying on one or two pillows, progressing to extension in prone-lying. The spine should be positioned so that it is straight with no lateral deviation. Pain relief in prone-lying may be due to a reduction in intradiscal pressure, an alteration in an anterior direction of the nucleus pulposus, the fact that the motion segment is not bearing weight, a reduction in venous congestion in the lumbar spine, or an alteration in the pH values around the nerve root.

In the standing position, as the lumbar spine moves into more extension, increased weight is taken by the apophyseal joints, and less through the discs, and this may be a factor in pain relief (*see* p. 30 for advice for these patients). Where there is disc space narrowing and subsequent overriding of facets with secondary arthrotic changes in the apophyseal joints, *hyper*extension often aggravates local back pain, and the patient would be better not to go to the extreme of this movement.

Pain relief using flexion

It may appear feasible that those patients who obtain relief from symptoms when in a flexed posture would automatically benefit from flexion exercises, but this is not always the case. Patients with discogenic pathology often stand with a flexion deformity, and may be comfortable initially curled up in bed. However, this position allows the nucleus to move posteriorly, so that when the patient then attempts to extend his spine, he is unable to do so — the flexion deformity is thus increased.

Using a flexion exercise for pain relief is effective only if the patient gets relief both during *and after* the exercise. Patients with a marked lordosis, early arthrosis, hypermobile backs or spondylolisthesis often benefit from a flexion regime. Where pain is exacerbated by postures or movements which involve the inner range of extension — prolonged standing, walking, reaching up to high shelves, painting the ceiling, etc. — a flexion exercise can be beneficial provided the patient learns how to use it functionally, i.e. during the otherwise-offending activity. (*see* Figs. 5.5, 5.8–11 and 5.16–17 for backward pelvic tilting and flexion exercises.)

Pain-relief using extension exercises

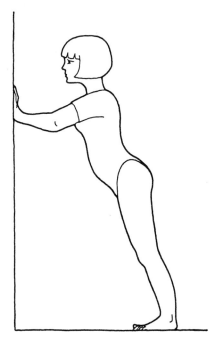

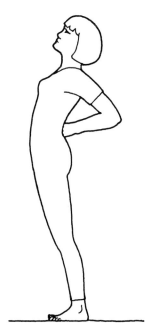

Fig. 5.6   Support hands on wall.
Let low back sag into
an arch.

Fig. 5.7   Stand with feet slightly
apart. Push hips
forwards, then
lean backwards.

Pain-relief using flexion

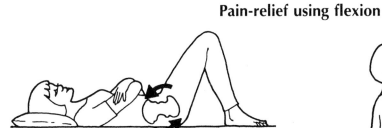

Fig. 5.8   Tilt pelvis backwards by
bracing abdominal muscles.

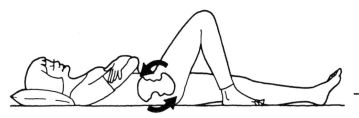

Fig. 5.9   Keep back flat and straighten
one leg, then the other.

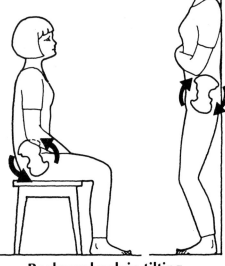

Backward pelvic tilting

Fig. 5.10
In sitting ...

Fig. 5.11
... and standing.

Stretching and Strengthening Exercises

Stretching and strengthening exercises are used to redress whatever imbalance is present, their ultimate purpose being to restore normal movement patterns. When performing these exercises, it is very important that strain is not imposed on another area of the spine. This applies particularly to the neck when exercises are given for the lumbar spine. The neck is vulnerable in (a) the 'sit-up' exercise used to strengthen the abdominal muscles, done with the hands behind the back of the head (Fig. 5.12) the tendency then being to pull the neck too far forward and strain it in an attempt to compensate for weak or fatigued abdominal muscles; and (b) extension exercises for the thoracic and lumbar spines when the neck is thrown back into extension (Fig. 5.13).

Sedentary workers who are chairbound for most of the day need to carry out stretching and strengthening exercises, activities or sports to offset the typical pattern of imbalance that occurs, as follows:

- *Tightness of*:   iliopsoas;
                     hamstrings;
                     erector spinae;
                     upper portion of trapezius and suboccipital muscles.
- *Weakness of*:   abdominals;
                     glutei;
                     quadriceps.
- *Dysfunction of*: thoracic and lumbar extension;
                     upper thoracic extension;
                     upper cervical flexion.

Stretching tight structures

Stretches should be applied slowly to a muscle until slightly beyond the point of comfort is reached, and then held for 8 seconds.

Iliopsoas stretch

The common method of stretching iliopsoas involves lying supine on a bed, with the muscle to be stretched extended by hanging that thigh over the side. Gravity-assisted stretching of the iliopsoas occurs. The opposite hip and knee should be flexed up to the chest to flatten the lumbar spine. An iliopsoas stretch can also be carried out effectively standing up with one foot on a stool and the tight hip extended until the patient feels the stretch in this hip (Fig. 5.14).

Hamstring stretch

One heel is placed on a stool with the affected knee straight. With both hands, the knee is held in extension and the hamstrings are stretched by leaning forwards from the hips. The lumbar spine should be kept straight during this procedure to stabilize the pelvis. Further stretch is gained by bending the knee of the supporting leg to increase hip flexion in the affected leg (Fig. 5.15).

Erector spinae stretch

The passive flexion stretch shown in Fig. 5.16 effectively stretches erector spinae. Some patients prefer to use the side-lying position (Fig. 5.17).

These exercises strain the neck and low back

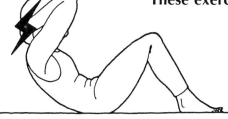

Fig. 5.12

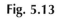

Fig. 5.13

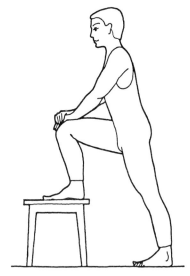

Fig. 5.14   Hip stretch. Lean forwards to feel a stretch in the hip of the weight-bearing leg.

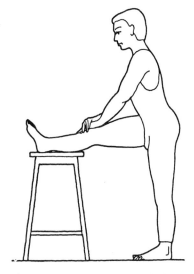

Fig. 5.15   Hamstring stretch: keep lumbar spine straight.

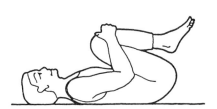

Fig. 5.16   Passive flexion stretch for back muscles.

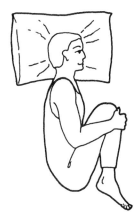

Fig. 5.17   Passive flexion stretch for back muscles – sometimes an easier position.

Stretch of upper portion of trapezius and suboccipital muscles

This all-important exercise is useful to prevent the forward head posture occurring (*see also* pp. 52–9).

Where head posture is already poor, the patient may have to start the exercise lying down with the head supported so as not to make the deformity worse (Fig. 5.18). The chin is first tucked in and, maintaining this, the head is pushed down into the supporting pillow/s. The patient is asked at the same time to feel his neck lengthening. The next stage is in the sitting or standing position. Again, the chin is tucked in and the head pushed backwards (perhaps against a wall), and the back of the head upwards. It is helpful for the patient to feel as if he is being lifted up from the crown of his head. A good time to practise this exercise is in the car when stopped at traffic lights: the head is pushed into the headrest (correctly positioned this should be level with the eyes).

The upper cervical spine should also be stretched in combination with cervical spine flexion—first upper, then the remainder of the cervical spine (Figs. 5.19, 5.20).

Strengthening exercises

Abdominal muscle strengthening

The patient must first learn how to *tilt the pelvis backwards* in the crook-lying position using the recti and oblique abdominal muscles (Fig. 5.8, p. 123). Some patients find this almost impossible to do at first; invariably these are the ones who benefit most from the exercise once they have mastered it.

The patient places his thumbs against the anterior superior iliac spines to give resistance to the movement (this brings in the oblique abdominals more effectively). He then attempts to flatten the lumbar spine against the supporting surface. If this proves difficult, he can imagine that he is putting on a pair of very tight jeans. The contraction is held for 10 seconds, initially to the expiratory phase of breathing, but later he should learn to breathe in and out gently while doing the exercise. Complete relaxation should follow each exercise.

Curl-downs (*see* Fig. 5.21)

These are a useful way of strengthening the abdominals in first inner and later middle range, as they avoid the tendency to push the head forwards that occurs when patients try to do 'sit-ups' from the crook-lying position. The feet should be kept flat on the supporting surface, but not anchored down, to minimize iliopsoas activity.

The patient sits up first, lightly holding on to both knees; then, flattening his low back and tucking in his chin, he slightly lowers his trunk, then returns to the starting position, helping with his hands if necessary. The exercise is progressed gradually by:

  not using the hands for assistance;
  lowering the trunk further and further (so long as he can return to the
    starting position);
  resting the hands on his shoulders;
  stopping for a count of 5 during the lowering part of the exercise and
    then lowering the trunk further before coming up again.

Neck stretches

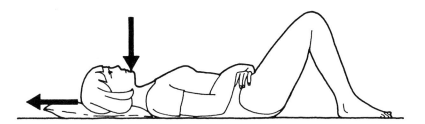

Fig. 5.18   Crook-lying is a useful position for gravity-assisted exercises for a weak neck. This posture correction exercise can later be progressed in the standing position (Fig. 5. 19).

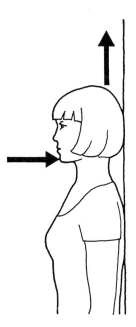

Fig. 5.19   Posture correction exercise: keeping chin in, push head backwards, lengthening the neck at the same time.

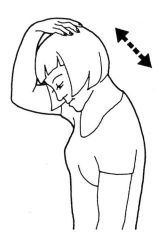

Fig. 5.20   Upper neck stretch.

Abdominal muscle strengthening: curl-downs

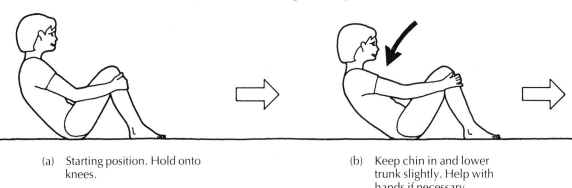

(a)   Starting position. Hold onto knees.

(b)   Keep chin in and lower trunk slightly. Help with hands if necessary.

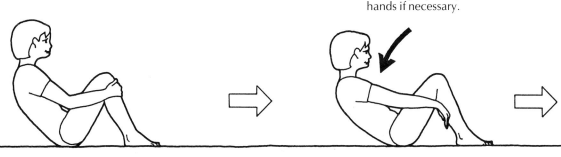

(c)   Up to starting position.

(d)   Now lower trunk slowly without using hands....

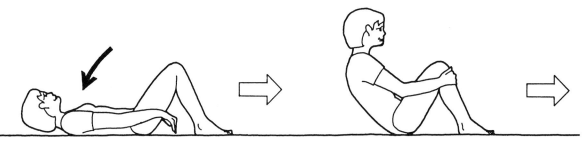

(e)   ...as the muscles get stronger, lower the trunk further...

(f)   ...always returning to starting position.

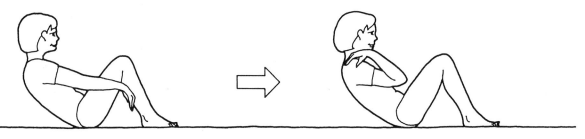

(g)   Progress by statically holding a position.

(h)   Then hold position, keeping hands on shoulders.

Fig. 5.21

Strengthening exercises for gluteal and quadriceps muscles

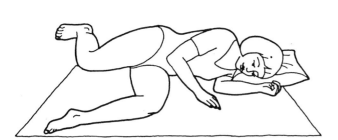

Fig. 5.22   Gluteal muscle strengthening –
starting position. Lift top leg
upwards and backwards.

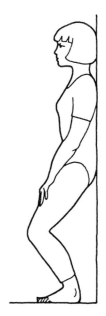

Fig. 5.24   Strengthening exercise
for knees: lower body
slightly into semisquat,
resting back against
wall.

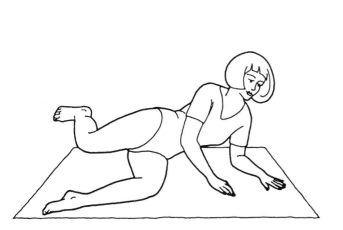

Fig. 5.23   A more advanced starting
position for strengthening
gluteal muscles.

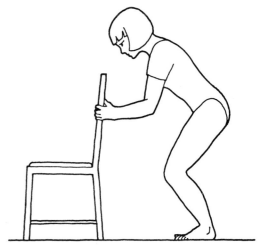

Fig. 5.25   The back stretch:
lengthen the back,
slowly lowering trunk
to semisquat position,
using chair for support.

Gluteal muscle strengthening

In side-lying with the underneath knee bent and the knee of the top leg also bent, the top leg is lifted upwards and then backwards (*see* Fig. 5.22), and then returned to the starting position. Progression is by a change of starting position to a more upright posture (*see* Fig. 5.23), using the underneath forearm for support.

Quadriceps muscle strengthening

The quadriceps are best strengthened for functional use by semisquats, not flexing the knees beyond 90°. These can be performed with the patient resting his back against a wall and slowly lowering his body in the posture correction exercise (*see* Fig. 5.24), with the back stretch (*see* Fig. 5.25), or in a swimming pool.

Stretches for Dysfunction

Stretches for thoracolumbar extension are shown in Figs. 5.1–5.4, 5.6, 5.7. Mid and upper thoracic extension can be gained by leaning backwards over the back of a roll with the hands behind the head (Fig. 5.26). An effective stretch for cervical flexion is shown in Fig. 5.20; this is contraindicated in the presence of recent discogenic pathology.

Easing Stiffness

People in sedentary occupations often complain of spinal stiffness. The compressive effects of sitting must be offset by frequent changes of position, walking and, ideally, swimming. A warm bath or standing with the back to a shower (Fig. 5.27) help the loosening-up process.

Exercises as part of a posture-re-education programme

Exercises alone are unlikely to correct a poor posture, but specific exercises can be usefully employed to gain range of movement, e.g. thoracic extension, lack of which may have been contributing to the poor posture. Strengthening muscle groups, such as the abdominals, will increase tone in them which will help to stabilize the lumbar spine in standing. Postural awareness must also be taught (*see* pp. 88–9, 100–2).

Sport

Theoretically, some form of sporting activity should be the answer to easing stiffness. Yoga, taught by a good teacher, is often helpful for hypermobile patients, because they are more comfortable when their joints are gently stretched, but not overstretched or held for too long at the end of range. Sports such as aerobics, rugby and jogging undoubtedly have other benefits in terms of health and relieving tension, but as far as the back and neck are concerned they tend to be too violent and jar the spine.

Swimming is the best sport, if the patient likes the water that is, but different strokes have different effects on the spine. The crawl is on the whole the best stroke; breaststroke tends to jerk the back into extension and people often swim with their heads out of the water placing the neck in too much extension. Often just floating on the back is helpful; the effect of buoyance provides a 'water' corset, and moving the limbs gently gives the back muscles exercise without loading the spine.

If the patient gets back pain during or after a particular sport, his technique should be checked to see if it could be improved.

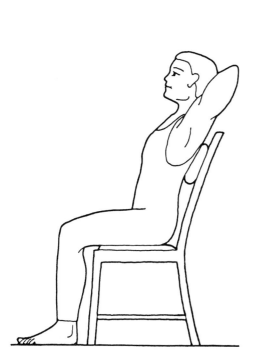

Fig. 5.26   Stretch for upper thoracic extension: lean backwards over a foam roll.

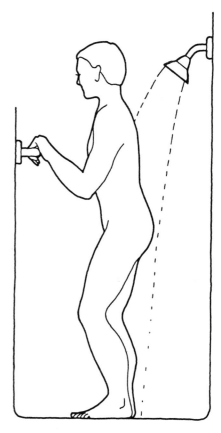

Fig. 5.27   A good way to loosen the back in the morning — stand with back to a hot shower.

6
Children and Teenagers

It may come as a surprise to learn that a significant number of children, and especially adolescents, get backache. A study carried out by Fairbank *et al.* in 1984 revealed that out of 446 schoolchildren aged 13–17, a quarter of them had a history of back pain. Relatively few children will complain of back pain to their doctors; most will cope by subconsciously fidgeting, tilting their chairs forward onto the front legs (Fig. 6.1), which is one means of straightening their backs to relieve discomfort, or assume what may appear to be unacceptable postures (Fig. 6.2). Back pain in children is often dismissed as being 'psychological' in origin.

Clinically, I see an increasing number of children, their main complaints being 'growing pains' (now recognized to be due predominantly to ligamentous strain caused by hypermobility, Beighton *et al.*, 1983), injury from falls, and aches and pains due to poor posture. This chapter deals mainly with trauma and postural problems, though many of these will also be associated with hypermobility.

Trauma

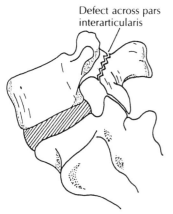

Defect across pars interarticularis

Fig. 6.3 Spondylolysis.

To some extent, falls and collisions are inevitable in the young. Little is known about the long-term effect on the spine of falls from, for instance, a climbing frame or horse, or of collisions during contact sports such as rugby, though it makes sense to have children playing such sports in size groups rather than age groups. Young intervertebral discs are sparsely innervated, and it is conceivable that they may sustain injury in the absence of symptoms.

The role of repeated trauma is considered to be a major factor in the development of a pars defect in spondylolysis (Fig. 6.3), certainly in the athlete (Jackson *et al.*, 1976). Repetitive jarring of the spine through landing heavily from badly-designed slides which are too steep to brake the descent (Figs. 6.4, 6.5) may well cause microtrauma to the spine, the effects of which may not cause symptoms until later in life. The child's spine is, indeed, more resilient than that of an adult, but that does not justify the unfortunate practice of placing toddlers on slides before they have the coordination to brake any impact by using their hands.

Postural Problems

Aches and pains of postural origin are initially due to ligamentous over-stretching. Uncomfortable in themselves, ligamentous strains deserve special attention, as they are often the precursor to discogenic problems (*see* p. 20) later in life.

Compare the alert posture of a four-year-old (Fig. 6.6) with that of an adolescent (Fig. 6.7) and you will see marked differences. By the mid-teens, habitual postures have started to cause structural changes in the skeleton and soft tissues, e.g. the upper round back deformity, absent in 11-year-olds, is evident in some 15-year-olds (Salminen, 1984). Very young children naturally adopt good working postures, so we must consider what can cause these to degenerate into unattractive slouches.

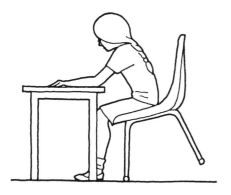

Fig. 6.1 Tilting chair forwards to get closer to work on table.

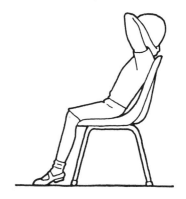

Fig. 6.2 Stretching back for comfort.

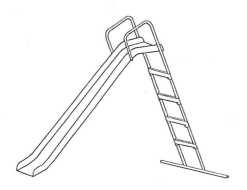

Fig. 6.4 Slope too steep → high impact landing.

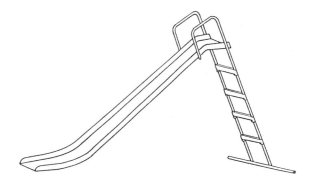

Fig. 6.5 Gentler slope with slide extension → less jarring.

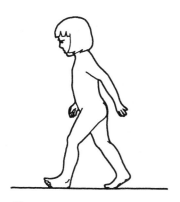

Fig. 6.6 Alert posture of a four-year-old child.

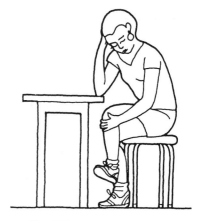

Fig. 6.7 Typical posture of an adolescent.

Youngsters are influenced by examples set by their family, teachers and peers as to what are acceptable postures. Therapists should be aware that they, too, act as role models to their patients. 'Do as I say, but not as I do' is certainly a recipe for non-compliance in this field.

Poor writing postures develop for many reasons: stress, fatigue, poor self-esteem, children hiding what they are writing from other children, badly designed furniture (*see below*), sitting for too long and lack of posture education in some primary schools. The time when the child starts to learn how to write is a critical period. Good or bad movement patterns start to be established, which soon become habitual. In the same way that the child's posture is important when, for example, playing tennis, so also is it important as he begins to write. To simply move a pencil across the page is not an exercise that demands a high level of muscular tension, yet children—and adults—can be seen to be gripping the pencil hard, their knuckles white with tension, shoulders hunched, neck twisted and the spine flexed (Fig. 6.8). The child has to be taught to prepare the body for writing, so that it is relaxed; this will then enable him to write using the minimum amount of energy necessary (Fig. 6.9). If a poor writing posture is allowed to develop, it can take a long time to correct, because the child gets used to writing using a particular posture, and then finds when it is corrected that it feels strange and his writing initially worsens.

Good teaching/learning strategies are necessary which are appropriate to the age of the children, e.g. using a problem-solving approach where the children work out efficient postures themselves, or using photographs and cuttings from magazines as a basis for discussing attractive postures. Particular problems are posed by tall children, especially girls, who attempt to reduce their height by rounding their backs, and young girls reaching puberty who are embarrassed by their developing breasts and adopt a similar slouched posture. A tactful and sensitive approach is essential.

Physical education lessons provide the ideal environment for correct posture, a good kinaesthetic sense and correct body-use to be taught. The results of a study (Handley, 1986) demonstrated that 8-year-old children badly misused their bodies during lifting, stooping, pushing and pulling in games and activities. There was excessive use of the lower back, little use of the leg muscles and a forward head posture.

PE lessons should redress the muscle imbalance that occurs with prolonged sitting postures (*see* p. 124). Overemphasis on flexion, e.g. forced toe-touching in the standing position (Fig. 6.10) or sit-ups with hands behind the head (Fig. 6.11) simply perpetuate the imbalance. Hamstrings are better stretched in the standing position with one foot on a bench (Fig. 6.12), bending from the hips with the back straight.

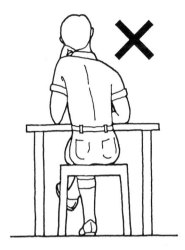

Fig. 6.8 Poor writing posture.

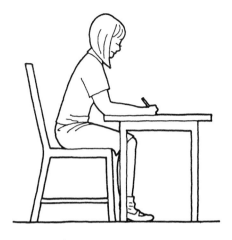

Fig. 6.9 Relaxed writing posture.

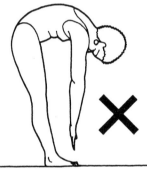

Fig. 6.10 *Forced* toe-touching can tear the hamstring muscles.

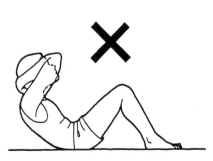

Fig. 6.11 Sit-ups with hands behind head encourage poor neck posture. Curl-downs (*see* Fig. 5.21, p. 128) are better.

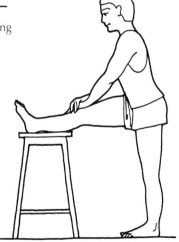

Fig. 6.12 A better way to stretch the hamstring muscles: keeping the back straight.

Instead of 'windmills' (Fig. 6.13), which combine flexing with rotation—a movement not to be encouraged because of its adverse effect on the discs (*see* p. 12)—a safer alternative is shown in Fig. 6.14. The abdominal muscles can be strengthened without bringing in the forward head posture depicted in Fig. 6.11 by the exercise described on p. 126 (Fig. 5.21). Bilateral straight-leg-raising from the floor is a dangerous exercise which puts excessive strain on the low back. Swimming is by far the best form of exercise because compression forces are low yet the antigravity muscles are exercised. Ideally, children of all ages should participate in some form of exercise daily, including walking to school where this is feasible. In schools where there is little provision for physical education, it is essential that the children participate in some form of exercise at the weekend, and swim after school.

Seating (*see also* Chapter 3)

Children are 4–5 cm taller today than they were in the last century, but furniture height has not increased proportionately. By the time the child reaches adolescence, most of his school day will be spent sitting. In one class there will be children of varying heights and measurements, so one standard chair will not suit all of them. Children who are taller or smaller than average are particularly disadvantaged: the tall child will automatically slouch, because of excessive hip flexion tilting the pelvis backwards, taking the lumbar spine into flexion (Fig. 6.15); the small child, with no foot support and a gap at the back of the seat will also slouch in order to obtain some stability (Fig. 6.16). Poor postural reflexes are then set up which very quickly become habitual, so that even when supplied with a suitable chair, the child will automatically slouch. It is now illegal for employers to provide unsuitable seating for office workers and, perhaps, one day the same will apply with regard to schoolchildren. Adjustable chairs would be ideal, but they are expensive. A simple improvement would be having chairs of differing heights in each classroom, but this would only work where the children sit facing the teacher. Where children work in groups, they could each have their own chair and carry it around, but teachers may understandably be concerned about the safety implications of this. Correct table height would also be unresolved.

The same situation regarding unsuitable seating tends to be perpetuated in the home (Fig. 6.17) even though chairs with adjustable seat and footrest heights are available for the 1–12 year olds (Fig. 6.18).

To some extent, spinal postural problems in young children are offset by the fact that they do not sit for as long a period as do adolescents, and run around a lot more. Physical education periods and other activities go some way towards compensating for the static position of sitting. With a reduction in physical education periods in some schools, however, this type of postural problem correspondingly increases.

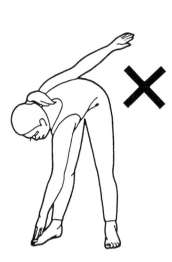

Fig. 6.13 Repetitive bending and twisting to one side stresses the discs.

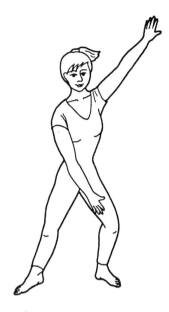

Fig. 6.14 A better stretch.

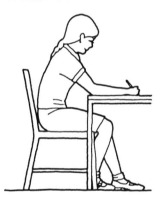

Fig. 6.15 Chair is too low.

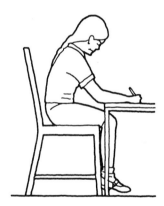

Fig. 6.16 Chair is too high — no foot support.

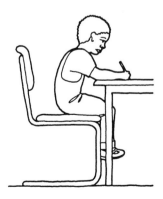

Fig. 6.17 Wrong size chair sets up poor balance reflexes.

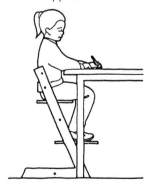

Fig. 6.18 Adjustable child's chair with foot support encourages spinal extension.

Desks

Just as chairs need to be of varying heights, so do desks. A desk which is too high will encourage poor posture especially in the neck (Fig. 6.19): a right-handed person tends to flex his head and neck laterally to the left side. A desk that is too low encourages slouching (Fig. 6.20). The relationship between chair and desk height is also important in that even if one is correct, e.g. correct chair height with incorrect desk height, the benefits of the correct piece of furniture are lost. Problems arise when the distance between the chair and desk is fixed as in some old-fashioned furniture because, while a gap allows easy access for the child, it prevents him getting close to the desk, thereby encouraging more bending forward.

Another important consideration is the angle of the writing surface. The distance between the child's eye and the reading material on the desk will vary depending on the size and clarity of the print, the child's eyesight and whether or not the light is good. One way of narrowing the distance between the reading material and the eyes is for the child to slouch. On straightening his spine, this distance is increased, even if the child is bending forwards from his hips. The working surface itself, therefore, has to be brought nearer to the eyes, and one way of doing this is to use a 10–15° slope (Fig. 6.21). Using a sloping surface is, of course, common practice for draughtsmen. The old desks in which the children kept their books and which had sloping surfaces have largely been replaced by tables with flat tops. Shortage of space is partly responsible for this; the tables need to be stackable so that the room can be used for different purposes. Also with teaching methods where the children work together in groups, the tables need to be light so that they are easy to move. The use of a writing slope* (which can be folded flat and stacked away when not in use, Fig. 6.22) with a 'lip' to prevent pens, etc. rolling off achieves the same effect as the old desks and is not expensive. Young children especially enjoy writing on one because it is more comfortable.

Posture when writing

Even with good seating, some effort is still required on the part of the child. Poor postural habits, once established, are difficult to remove. If it is accepted practice for a child in primary school to sit with his head flexed and rotated, shoulders hunched and trunk asymmetrical, this will become an established pattern of movement. This bad habit will then feel right to the child and, consequently, any attempts to correct it will feel wrong. The tense, rigid posture reminiscent of the Victorian age is, of course, undesirable, but it is essential that the child is frequently reminded by the teacher to adopt a natural and relaxed posture, bending from the hips rather than the waist when writing.

* Obtainable from Back Care, 151 Gwydir Street, Cambridge, CB1 2LJ. Tel: 0223-351933.

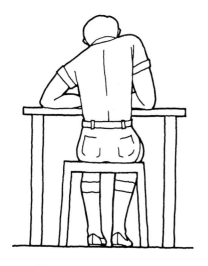

Fig. 6.19 Desk is too high.

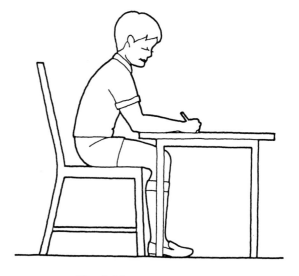

Fig. 6.20 Desk is too low.

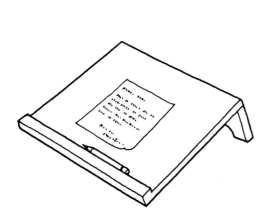

Fig. 6.22 Detail of writing slope.

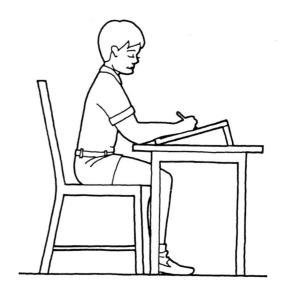

Fig. 6.21 Use of writing slope encourages good posture.

Carrying

The best way to carry heavy textbooks is in a rucksack over both shoulders (Fig. 6.23) to encourage symmetry, but even so the load must be kept within reason. Lockers with a large storage capacity should be provided to minimize the number of books the child has to carry around with him. Asymmetrical postures result from carrying heavy single bags (Fig. 6.24) or single strap satchels over a hunched-up shoulder (Fig. 6.25). Balance can be achieved by placing the strap over the opposite shoulder, which also frees both hands (Fig. 6.26).

Variations in Ranges of Movement

The range of movement in children's joints varies considerably. At both ends of the movement spectrum are those with naturally stiffer joints (i.e. hypomobile types) and those with lax ligaments, and subsequent loose backs (hypermobility). Children who are naturally stiff-jointed will loosen up to some extent with exercise, but can never achieve the range of movement of those who are naturally hypermobile, and should not be pressurized into forcing movements. Stiffer-jointed children also have less 'spring' in their joints. The secondary school physical education teacher may be aware of these natural variations in range, but not necessarily the primary school teacher unless PE is his main subject.

Hypermobile children often excel at gymnastics for obvious reasons: their excessive range of spinal movement enables them to perform movements which are impossible for their stiffer peers, e.g. the crab, back and front walkovers. There is a danger in these children, in particular if they perform these movements excessively without sufficient time allowed for recovery. Trauma can result in localized areas of stiffness, which then puts stress on already hypermobile joints causing recurrent backache, invariably localized to the low lumbar spine.

References

Beighton P., Grahame R., Bird H. (1983). *Hypermobility of Joints*. Berlin, Heidelberg: Springer-Verlag.

Fairbank J. C. T., Pynsent P. B., Van Poorliet J. A., Phillips H. (1984). Influence of anthropometric factors and joint laxity in the incidence of adolescent back pain. *Spine* **9**, 461.

Handley J. (1986). 1933 and all that? *Bul. Phys. Ed.*, **22**, 12.

Jackson D. W., Wiltse L., Cirincione R. (1976). Spondylolysis in the female gymnast. *Clin. Orthop. and Rel. Res.*, **117**, 68.

Salminen J. J. (1984). The adolescent back. A field study of 370 Finnish schoolchildren. *Acta Paediatrica Scandinavica Supp.*, **315**, 1.

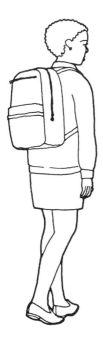

Fig. 6.23   A rucksack over both
shoulders encourages
symmetrical posture.

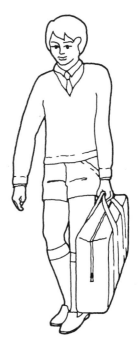

Fig. 6.24   Asymmetrical
posture.

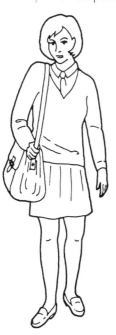

Fig. 6.25   Asymmetrical posture: hunched-up
shoulder.

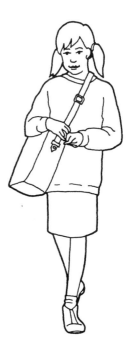

Fig. 6.26   Single strap satchels should be
carried with the strap over the
opposite shoulder.

7
Pregnancy

Few women escape some type of backache/pain during pregnancy or postpartum, yet it receives scant attention compared with the overwhelming interest in the fetus and baby. In approximately 50% of pregnant women, the pain is of sufficient intensity and duration to affect their lifestyle in some way, and a third of these women experience severe pain (Mantle *et al.*, 1977, 1981; Fast *et al.*, 1987; Berg *et al.*, 1988). Nevertheless, some women who have suffered from backache before pregnancy are occasionally surprised to find that it is no worse, and indeed sometimes less during pregnancy, possibly due to the 'strut' effect; others report increased pain.

Causes of Backache in Pregnancy and Postpartum

Hormonal influence on collagen tissue

An increase in progesterone and relaxin levels causing relaxation of ligaments starts early in pregnancy and increases during the last three months. Collagen in the ligaments is replaced by a modified form that is more extensible, and this allows more movement in the pelvic joints to accommodate the growing fetus. At the same time, however, the ligaments are more susceptible to being strained, those of the *sacroiliac joints* (Fig. 7.1) being most prone. Overriding of a sacroiliac joint can also occur when it becomes locked in a new position. As the ligaments return to their normal condition postpartum, which takes up to five months after delivery (Abramson *et al.*, 1934), the malaligned joint can cause overstretching of ligaments giving rise to symptoms, sometimes from the opposite sacroiliac joint which is under strain. Areas of pain referral are shown in Figs. 7.2, 7.3. However, pain over the sacroiliac joints or tenderness on palpation does not necessarily implicate the underlying joints, and a thorough examination should always be carried out to see if the pain is, in fact, referred from higher in the spine. Marked ligamentous laxity can also cause widening of the symphysis pubis in some pregnant women, often in association with lax sacroiliac joints, giving incapacitating pain over the symphysis pubis when walking, radiating into the medial aspects of the thighs.

Ligamentous laxity also causes an *accentuation of the thoracic and lumbar curves*. Thoracic pain is fairly common because of the increasing weight of the breasts, combined with ligamentous laxity, and poor posture when breastfeeding or changing nappies. Towards term, the flaring of the ribs can cause strain at the costovertebral or costotransverse joints. The increased lumbar lordosis, imposing a greater load on the lumbar apophyseal joints, can also cause symptoms.

Additionally during this period of ligamentous laxity, the modified collagen, because of its higher water content and greater volume, can cause pressure on pain-sensitive structures.

Ligamentous laxity is greater in the second pregnancy than in the first, but does not increase further with subsequent pregnancies. It is also greater in twin pregnancies than in singleton pregnancies.

Increased weight

The increasing size and weight of the fetus imposes greater stress on the spine, not only in standing and sitting, but also in lying positions.

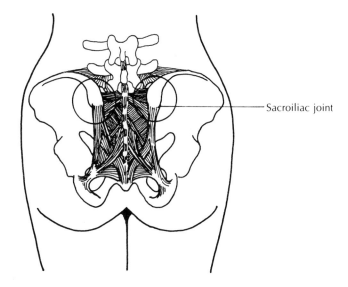

Fig. 7.1

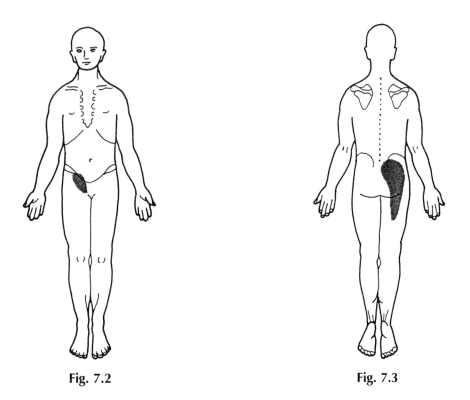

Fig. 7.2   Fig. 7.3

Areas of pain from sacroiliac joint

Altered mechanics

The increase in the lumbar and thoracic curves of the mother-to-be together with the distending abdomen causes a marked change in posture and body mechanics. Certain movements are awkward and the mother-to-be becomes more accident-prone.

Fatigue

This can be overwhelming, especially in the early months of pregnancy and after delivery. Compounded with anxiety about the fetus/new baby, this can have a detrimental effect on posture.

During and after labour

If the lithotomy position is used for delivery or perineal repair, especially when careless placing or removing of the legs in the stirrups has occurred, back strain may result. Epidural haematomas can also occur in the venous plexus of the epidural space. These thin-walled veins could be torn by a sudden increase in intravenous pressure (Scott et al., 1976). It is conceivable that ensuing dural adhesions could later give rise to signs and symptoms of adverse neural tension.

Poor ergonomics

The amount of bending and lifting the new mother has to do day and night is legion and puts her spine at considerable risk. Previously safe movements become hazardous because they are done repetitively.

Prevention

A significant amount of the pain associated with pregnancy can be prevented, or its severity reduced (Mantle et al., 1981) through education given at the appropriate time. Generally, women are less receptive after the birth than before because of increased fatigue and preoccupation with the baby, so it is imperative that the new mother-to-be is seen by the physiotherapist early in her pregnancy as well as postpartum.

Advice on the purchase of suitable equipment

This can be offered to prevent excessive back strain after the baby is born. Attention should be focused on the items which will be used most frequently.

Prams and buggies

When choosing a pram or buggy, the mother's lifestyle has to be taken into account. If she is going to be pushing it around a lot in country lanes, one with an efficient wheel system where the front wheels can swivel is preferable as it makes the buggy much easier to push. To compare buggies, the mother should load one with, say, a full shopping bag, to see how easy it is to push. If she is going to be lifting the buggy in and out of cars or on and off buses a lot, then a light-weight buggy would be more practical. Handles should be the correct height to avoid stooping: tall women in particular should be careful about this (Figs. 7.4, 7.5). The mother should push the buggy forwards and check if she has to stoop to do so, rather than deciding on the height from a position with her elbows into her side. A head support pillow in the pram, buggy or car seat is good for the baby's posture, and prevents the head falling into extreme lateral flexion (Fig. 7.6).

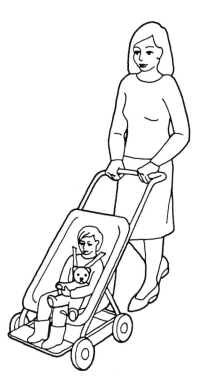

Fig. 7.4 Handles of buggy:
correct height.

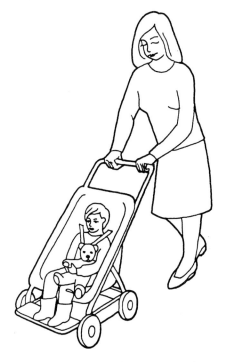

Fig. 7.5 Handles of buggy are too low
for tall mothers.

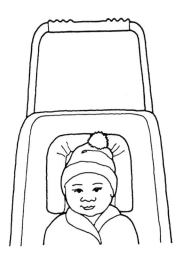

Fig. 7.6 Support of baby's neck.

Cots

A dropside cot is a help to avoid some flexion strain. Twisting to lift should be avoided by standing at a diagonal (Fig. 7.7). If the mother-to-be has previously had backache, it might be worth her considering a cot which has two levels for the baby—a higher one for the young baby and a lower one for use when the child can stand up in the cot. A cot is not the ideal place in which to change the baby's nappy, and it is a pity that this practice is encouraged in some maternity hospitals.

Baby baths

Baby baths on low stands, that involve lots of carrying of water in jugs in order to fill them, or involve lifting and lowering when full of water, should be avoided unless the father can do the carrying. There is nothing wrong with having a special washing up bowl reserved for the baby, placed on the draining board, or bathing the baby in the sink (Fig. 7.8). Alternatively, baby baths can be bought which can be filled directly from the bath taps and emptied into the bath by a plug; these can rest over the bath so that the mother can kneel alongside.

Carrycots

All carrycots are a problem because their centre of gravity is at a distance from the carrier's body even when the carrycot is held up close to it. They have largely been superseded by car seats which are more compact and are an easier load to carry. If carrycots must be used, the mother should be able to keep her forearm close to her (Fig. 7.9) rather than hold the centre of the handle, and should carry it in front of her body not to the side (Fig. 7.10). A 'Moses' basket is a lot lighter but is, of course, less protective. A sling may be preferred (*see* p. 154).

Correct lifting techniques

These need to be practised until they become second nature. If education is left until too late in the pregnancy, the quadriceps may be too weak to cope with the heavier load, and it may be physically impossible for the mother-to-be to lift properly (Polden and Mantle, 1990). The distended abdomen prevents loads being held close to the centre of the body, incurring an additional leverage problem. Women who are naturally hypermobile often tend to lock their knees into extension when bending to lift and make use of their greater-than-average range of spinal flexion. They in particular need checking and regular reinforcement throughout the pregnancy. Posters and videos in clinic waiting areas educating mothers-to-be about back care serve as useful reminders, as well as antenatal classes. The swimming pool is the ideal place to practise semisquats (Fig. 7.11) to strengthen the knees, but there is no substitute for repetitively practising correct lifting techniques in a coordinated manner. Heavy lifting should be avoided during the period of ligamentous laxity. This is not always easy when the pregnant woman already has a toddler demanding attention.

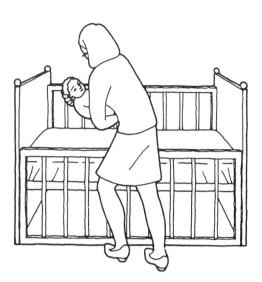

Fig. 7.7   Keep back as straight as possible. Avoid twisting by standing at a diagonal.

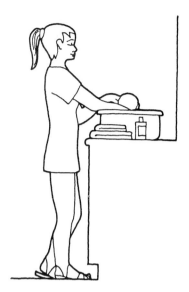

Fig. 7.8   Bathing baby on draining board — unorthodox, but good for mother's back.

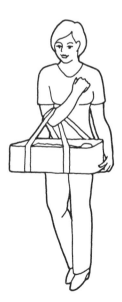

Fig. 7.9   Least stressful way of carrying a carrycot. Hold forearm close to body.

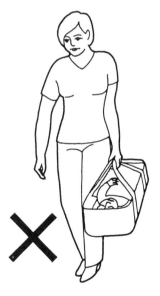

Fig. 7.10   Asymmetrical posture.

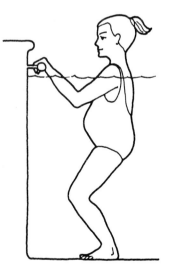

Fig. 7.11   Pool exercises are useful for strengthening knees.

Comfortable resting positions

Many women experience fatigue during pregnancy and often feel guilty about resting. They should be encouraged to have rest periods rather than fight the fatigue and, if they have other young children, seek help from family, friends or neighbours. Comfortable resting positions are shown in Figs. 7.12–7.18.

General activities

As far as possible, low-down activities should be performed from the kneeling position, e.g. bedmaking, cleaning the bath or attending to small children. Standing and leaning over work surfaces can cause ligamentous backache, which can often be prevented by placing one foot on a low stool or on the ledge under the sink. Periodically stretching the spine into extension also helps some women. Later in pregnancy as balance becomes more unstable, it is inadvisable to stand on high stools or climb step-ladders.

Exercise

Intensive exercise in pregnancy carries a risk to the fetus, and to the mother-to-be's ligaments, because of increased laxity, jerky and bouncy movements being particularly hazardous to the sacroiliac ligaments. On the other hand, physically fit women recover more rapidly after the birth than those who spend a less active pregnancy, so obviously some exercise is beneficial. General exercises such as walking, swimming and cycling are helpful. If cycling on roads is impractical because of heavy traffic, a static bicycle is a useful alternative as it provides excellent partial weight-bearing activity. Swimming is the safest exercise to improve general muscle tone (*see* 'Swimming Through Your Pregnancy' by Jane Katz under 'Further Reading') and group aqua-exercise classes are held in many swimming pools.

Gentle pelvic tilting should be taught in pregnancy, and practised in crook-lying, side-lying, prone-kneeling and standing. Only when it can be performed easily in the standing position should posture re-education be attempted. Pelvic tilting can relieve backache in some mothers-to-be, and it also makes them realize the importance of maintaining some tone in their abdominal muscles. If practised after the birth, so that the abdominal muscles are strong, this makes the back less vulnerable, together with enhanced appearance!

Abdominal muscle contractions should be taught in order for them to be practised eventually in functional positions, e.g. standing, while waiting in a queue. However motivated the mother-to-be may be, she is often unable to find time for herself after the birth. The exercises must somehow be fitted into her busy day, if necessary when she is having a bath or breastfeeding the baby. Initially, however, the exercises should be taught in crook-lying. It is more efficient to initiate a contraction during expiration, not inspiration. Using both thumbs over the anterior superior iliac spines to resist the movement encourages a stronger contraction of the oblique abdominals. If the mother has obvious difficulty in initiating an abdominal contraction postdelivery, it may be easier for her in the side-lying position because the abdomen protrudes and sags sideways and the muscle fibres are in their outer to middle range—their predelivery state (Polden and Mantle, 1990).

Comfortable resting postures

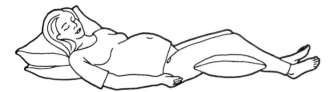

Fig. 7.12

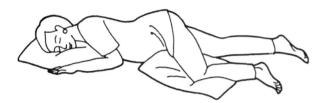

Fig. 7.13

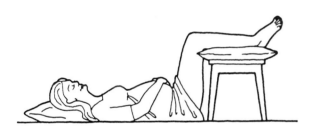

Fig. 7.14

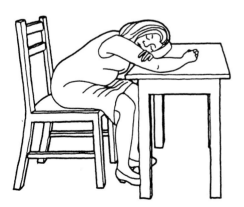

Fig. 7.15

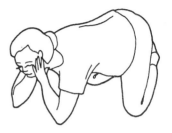

Fig. 7.16

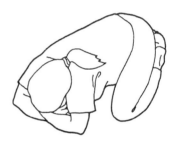

Fig. 7.17

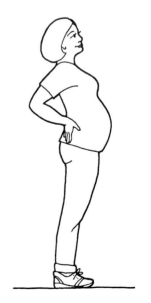

Fig. 7.18

Posture

During pregnancy, the centre of gravity in the standing position moves forward, and the spinal curves tend to become accentuated causing discomfort. The mother-to-be usually has to be taught to reduce these curvatures by:

> stretching up the back of the head;
> lifting up through the rib cage and relaxing back the shoulders, letting the arms roll outwards;
> tilting the pelvis backwards with abdominal and gluteal muscle contraction, so that she feels the baby sitting in the pelvis. The knees will automatically tend to bend slightly;
> lifting the weight from the medial arches of the feet and redistributing evenly through the feet.

Nappy changing

To begin with, the mother will probably be changing the baby's nappy up to 12 times a day. Prolonged stooping combined with ligamentous laxity and fatigue present a well-known hazard. Using a surface which is waist-high is ideal, or half kneeling on the floor rather than kneeling (Figs. 7.19–7.21) with all the necessary items in front to avoid twisting. The experienced mother will be able to change the nappy on her lap.

Breastfeeding

Comfort for the mother is essential during this important activity; indeed, the success of breastfeeding may depend on it. Slouched positions cause thoracic strain and the mother should get into the habit of first making sure that her back is supported (Fig. 7.22) and then bringing the baby to her, supported at a comfortable height on pillows, cushions or anything else that is to hand. A stool (or box, books, coffee table, etc.) to support the feet is often a help, as it encourages the mother to lean back and support her spine. Side-lying in bed is a very comfortable position for some mothers (Fig. 7.23).

Slings

Carrying the baby in a sling either in front (before the baby has head control) or on the mother's back (after the baby has head control) solves the problem of leverage presented by the carrycot and has the advantage of leaving the mother's hands free. The design of the sling should allow the mother to do it up herself unaided, and the material from which it is made should enable the baby to be slid into it. Some corduroy-type fabrics makes this a difficult and frustrating exercise. Slings to carry the baby on the front should be worn as high up as possible and should be tightly fixed to the mother (Fig. 7.24). It is often more comfortable for the mother to give extra support with her forearms under the sling. However, even tiny babies weigh a lot more when carried for any length of time, and because the baby is effectively 'lighter' in a sling than in a carrycot, mothers fall into the trap of carrying the child for too long.

Unless the mother is extremely fit, it is more sensible for her to use a sling for short periods and a pram for longer shopping trips; she is then not tempted to carry both child and shopping together.

Nappy changing

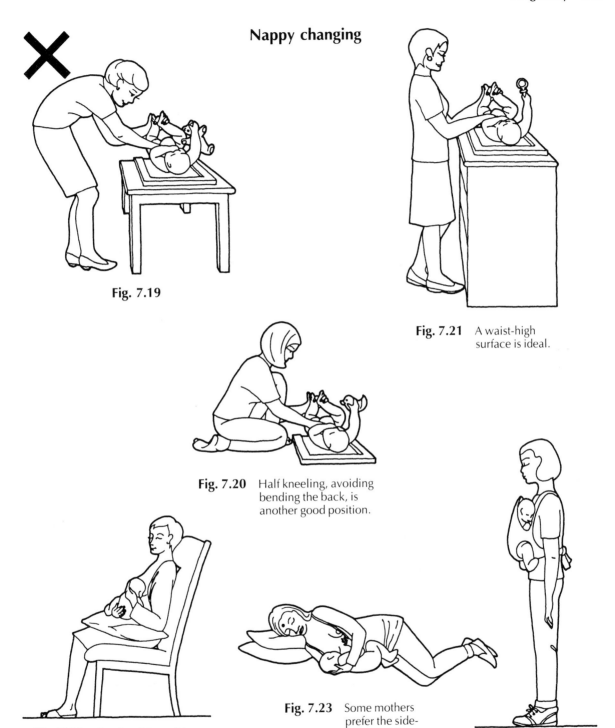

Fig. 7.19

Fig. 7.21   A waist-high
surface is ideal.

Fig. 7.20   Half kneeling, avoiding
bending the back, is
another good position.

Fig. 7.22   Comfortable position:
support in low back
and baby on pillow.

Fig. 7.23   Some mothers
prefer the side-
lying position.

Fig. 7.24   Wear sling as
high as possible,
and fix straps
tightly.

Breast feeding positions

Sacroiliac joint dysfunction   The sacroiliac joints are most frequently strained during pregnancy or postpartum. Careful assessment must, of course, always be carried out and if malalignment of joint surfaces is diagnosed, the appropriate manoeuvres should be carried out by the physiotherapist. In many cases, however, there is no 'bone out of place', the ligaments having been overstretched and muscle spasm accentuating the problem. A few days' rest or cutting down of activities often helps relieve pain. Fraser (1976) described a self-help manoeuvre for relieving sacroiliac pain (Fig. 7.25) which can be used once or twice a day to encourage the ilium and sacrum to remain in more normal correlation. For the left sacroiliac joint, the patient lies supine with the right leg straight; with her left hand she holds the left flexed knee at the level of the tibial tubercle and with her right hand cups the left heel so that the hip is in lateral rotation. The left knee is gently pulled to a point just lateral to the right shoulder and the left foot eased toward the right groin. The pull is then released and reapplied once or twice. The manoeuvre should then be performed on the opposite side. Figure 7.26 shows a comfortable resting position for relieving pain from the sacroiliac left joint.

Mothers-to-be who are prone to sacroiliac strains or malalignment often get relief from wearing a pelvic binder (see Fig. 7.27 for correct way to wear one) or a double layer of tubigrip (Fig. 7.28) with a hole cut in the middle. They should try to minimize asymmetrical stress on the pelvis such as occurs when carrying a child on the hip (Figs 7.29, 7.30), sitting on the floor with the legs curled to one side, and should get out of cars carefully, keeping both knees together and swinging out both legs together first.

References

Abramson V., Roberts S. M., Wilson P. D. (1934). Relaxation of the pelvic joints in pregnancy. *Surg. Gynecol. Obstet.*, **58**, 595.

Berg G., Hammar M., Möller-Nielsen J. *et al.* (1988). Low back pain during pregnancy. *Obst. Gynec.* **71**, 71.

Fast A., Shapiro D., Ducommun E. J., *et al.* (1987). Low back pain in pregnancy. *Spine*, **12**, 368.

Fraser D. (1976). Postpartum backache; a preventable condition? *Can. Fam. Phys.*, **22**, 1434.

Mantle M. J., Greenwood R. M., Currey H. L. F. (1977). Backache in pregnancy. *Rheum. Rehab.*, **16**, 95.

Mantle M. J., Greenwood R. M., Currey H. L. F. (1981). Backache in pregnancy. II: Prophylactic influence of backache classes. *Rheum. Rehab.*, **20**, 227.

Polden M., Mantle J. (1990). Physiotherapy in Obstetrics and Gynaecology. Oxford: Butterworth-Heinemann.

Scott B. B., Quisling R. G., Miller C. *et al.* (1976). Spinal epidural haematoma. *J. Am. Med. Ass.*, **235**, 513.

Further Reading

Katz J. (1985). *Swimming through your Pregnancy*. Wellingborough: Thorsons.

Relieving pain from sacroiliac joint

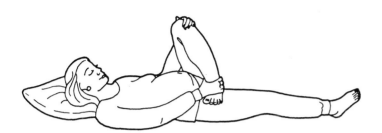

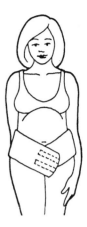

Fig. 7.25 A self-help manoeuvre for the left sacroiliac joint. Gently pull left knee towards right shoulder, and left foot towards right groin.

Fig. 7.27 Pelvic binder worn *under* abdomen.

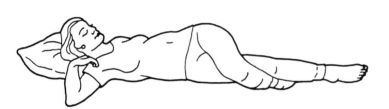

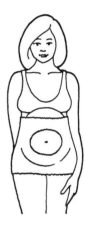

Fig. 7.26 Comfortable resting position for left sacroiliac joint.

Fig. 7.28 Double layer of tubigrip with hole cut in the middle.

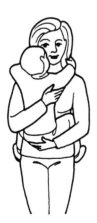

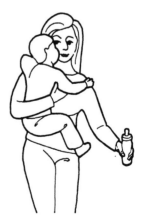

Fig. 7.29 Correct way to carry a child.

Fig. 7.30 Avoid asymmetrical stresses such as this!

Index

abdominal muscles 8, 116
    bracing exercises 120(*fig*)
    exercises during pregnancy 152
    strengthening 126, 128(*figs*)
activity/rest balance xiv
acute neck, temporary measures to
        support 70
adolescent *see* teenager
ankylosing spondylitis 42
antalgic postures 96, 97, 99(*figs*)
Alexander, F. M. xiv
apophyseal joint *see* vertebral
        column, apophyseal (facet) joint;
        see also facet syndrome

baby
    equipment, back-friendly 148–50
        correct sling use 154
    neck/head support 148
babycare posture 148–57
bed
    choice 64
    getting in/out 72, 73(*figs*)
    hotel 72
    improvement 62
bed-making 72
bedrest 72–5
    24-hour a day 74–5
    when inappropriate 75
bending 23(*figs*), 104
    backward 11(*fig*)
    forward 11(*fig*)
    turning and 13(*fig*)
breastfeeding posture 154, 155(*figs*)
brittle bones (osteoporosis) 42, 44

carrying
    by child/teenager 143(*figs*)
    childcare-related 150, 154–6
cervical flexion 56, 57(*figs*), 127(*fig*),
        130

cervical headaches 54, 55(*figs*)
cervicothoracic junction, pain 56
chair
    adjustable 86, 138
    armrests 82
    backrest 78
    choice 78
    desk height in relation to 82
    for:
        VDU operator 85(*fig*), 86
        child/teenager 138–40
    lumbar support 30, 41(*fig*), 78,
        79(*fig*)
    seat
        angle 80
        depth 82
        firmness 80
        height 80
        space under 82
        wedge to level 90
    see also sitting
child/teenager, backcare 134–42
    carrying 140, 143(*figs*)
    desks 140
    lifting, training for 112
    physical education 136–9
    postural problems 134–8
    sitting/seating 86, 138–40
    trauma effect 134
    writing poture 136, 137(*figs*),
        139–41
childcare posture 148–57
computer use *see* VDU (visual display
        unit) use
curl-downs 126, 128(*figs*)

desks 82, 140
double-jointed 24
driving 90
dynamic/static muscle work
        comparison xii

erector spinae stretch   124
exercises   120–30
  abdominal   120(*fig*), 126, 128(*figs*)
    pregnancy, during   152
  for:
    easing stiffness   130
    facet syndrome recovery   34
    pain relief   121(*figs*), 122–3
    posture re-education
        programme   130
  general principles   122
  gluteal   129(*figs*)–30
  hamstring   124, 136
  neck   56, 86, 126
  quadriceps   129(*fig*)–30
  when not to prescribe   120
extension   10, 121(*figs*), 122

facet syndrome   32–7
  areas of pain   32, 33(*fig*)
  backcare   32–6
  comfortable
      sitting/resting   36–7(*figs*)
  pain-relieving standing
      postures   35(*fig*)
  see also vertebral column,
      apophyseal (facet) joints
flat back   94, 95(*fig*)
flexion   10
  deformity   96, 97(*fig*)
    fixed   70
  for pain relief   122
forward head
    posture/syndrome   52–8
  aggravating factors   58
  causes   52, 53(*figs*)
  effect on:
    joints   52, 54
    movements   54
    muscles/soft tissues   54
  muscular pain   56

gibbus   46
growing pains   24, 134

hamstring stretch exercises   124, 136
headache   54
heel pad   50
hollow back   2, 94
hypermobility/hypermobility
    syndrome   xiii, 24
  in children   134

iliopsoas stretch exercise   124
insoles, cushioned   98
interspinous ligament ruptures   6, 22
intervertebral disc   4
  cross-section   7(*figs*)

degeneration   12, 32(*figs*)
  intradiscal pressure   4 in:
    driving   90
    sitting   94
    standing   94
    various muscle strengthening
        exercises   31(*fig*)
    various positions   31(*fig*)
  pathology   26
  posterior radial fissure   26
  posterolateral radial fissures   10
  prolapse   26
    recovery   30
    site of pain   28
    stages leading to   28
  sudden trauma   26
  syndromes   26–30
    hereditary predisposition to   26
ischial tuberosities   88

joints
  apophyseal *see* vertebral column,
      apophyseal (facet) joint
  end of range positions   xiii–xiv
  midtarsal   102
  range of movement   xii–xiii
  sacroiliac *see* sacroiliac joint
  subtalar   50, 102

kneeling stool   34, 80
kyphosis   42–5

lateral flexion   12, 98
  flexion deformity combined
      with   98
  rotation with   98
leaning forwards   104
leverage   108
lift/lifting   108–17
  childcare-related   150
  disc damage in relation to   26
  disc pressure in relation to   31(*fig*)
  leverage   108
  load position   112
  foot positioning   114
  grip   114
  ligament damage in relation to   22
  patient fitness for   116
  planning lift   114
  pregnancy/postpartum during   150
  safe, individual capacity
      for   110–12
  training for   112
ligament   6
  hypermobility   24
  interspinous ruptures   6
  laxity, degree of   xii–xiii, 142
    pregnancy/postpartum
        during   146

ligament (*cont.*)
  sprain/tear   22
  standing posture effect on   94
  strain   26, 134
    chronic ligamentous, of vertebral
        column posterior
        ligaments   20
    syndromes   20–4
long, round back   94
lordosis   40, 93(*fig*), 98
  increased   146
lumbar support–*see* chair
lying   62–75

mechanoreceptors   61
muscles
  abdominal *see* abdominal muscles
  back extensors   8
  gluteal   102, 116, 129(*figs*)–30
  hamstring, stretch exercise   124,
      136
  iliopsoas, stretch exercise   124
  paravertebral   116
  quadriceps   116, 129(*figs*)–30
  small, deep back   8
  static/dynamic work compared   xii
muscle spasm   8, 58

nappy changing posture   154
neck
  acute, temporary measures to
      support   70
  baby's support for   148
  exercises   126
  posture/comfort   66
  relaxation techniques   8, 58
nerve(s)   6–8
  areas of pain   15, 17(*figs*), 29
  compression   6–8, 14, 28
  root supply   16(*table*)
  sinuvertebral   8

orthosis   34, 50, 102
osteochondrosis
    (Scheuermann's)   42–4
osteoporosis   42, 44

pain   14
  from:
    apophyseal joints   32, 33(*figs*)
    lumbar curves   146
    nerve root disorders   15(*figs*),
        17(*figs*), 29(*figs*)
    sacroiliac joint   146, 147(*figs*)
    sitting   76
    standing   102
    thoracic curves   146
  referred   15(*figs*), 33(*figs*)

pelvic binder   156
pelvic tilting   34, 38, 120–2
pillows   66, 70
  butterfly   71(*fig*)
postpartum *see*
    pregnancy/postpartum backcare
posture   61–104
  re-education programme   130
pregnancy/postpartum,
    backcare   146–56
  backache
    causes   146–8
    prevention   148–56
  exercise   152
  posture   154–5
    breastfeeding   154
    nappy changing   154
    sling use   154
  resting positions   152, 153(*figs*)
  sacroiliac joint dysfunction   156

relaxation techniques, neck   8, 58
rest/activity balance   xiv
rotation   12
  with lateral flexion   12, 98

sacralization   26, 27(*fig*)
sacroiliac joint
  dysfunction during
      pregnancy/postpartum   38,
      156
  pain   146
sacroiliac syndromes   38
Scheuermann, H. W.   42
Scheuermann's osteochondrosis   42
Schmorl's nodes   4, 26, 42
Schroth, Katharina   48
sciatic list   96, 97(*fig*)
scoliosis   46–8
  corrective exercises   48, 49(*figs*)
  in children   46
  non-structural   46
  structural   46
sedentary worker, exercises   124
senile osteoporosis   42
short leg   26, 50
sinuvertebral nerve   8
sitting   76–82
  chair use, *see* chair
  child/teenager   138–40
  correction of posture   88, 89(*figs*)
  desk at   82, 140
  driving-related   90
  unsupported   76
sitting bones (ischial tuberosities)   88
skeletal types   94–5
sleeping positions   64–9
slipped disc   26

spinal stenosis 8, 9(*figs*)
spine *see* vertebral column (spine)
spondylolisis 26
    pars defect development 134
spondylolisthesis 26
sport 130
standing 92–105
    antalgic posture 96, 97(*figs*)
    asymmetrical 97(*fig*)
    cushioned insoles use 98
    effect on:
        apophyseal joints 94
        intradiscal pressure 94
        ligaments 94
        muscle activity 94
        vertebral column 92–4
    flexion deformity 96
        lateral flexion deformity
            combined with 98
    heel height effect on 98
    idealized posture 92
    lateral flexion with rotation 98
    pain produced by 102
    posture correction 100–2
    sciatic list 96
static/dynamic muscle work
        comparison xii
suboccipital/trapezius stretch
        exercise 56, 126
swimming 30, 58, 130

teenager *see* child/teenager, backcare
thoracic curves, pain 146
thoracic extension 130
trapezius/suboccipital stretch
        exercise 126
tropism 26
turning 13(*figs*)

upper round back 94

VDU (visual display unit) use 84–7
    chair choice 86
    exercises for operator 87(*figs*)

musculoskeletal disorder
        prevention 84
    regulations, European community
        directive-initiated 86
    sitting posture 85(*fig*), 88–9
vertebral column (spine)
    apophyseal (facet) joint 6, 8, 102
        referred pain from 32, 33(*figs*)
        standing posture effect on 94
        see also facet syndrome
    chronic posterior ligament
        strain 20
    compression on 12
    curves 2, 3(*figs*)
    extension 10, 121(*figs*), 123(*figs*)
    flexion 10
        cervical 130
        deformity 96, 98
        for pain relief 122
    interspinous ligament ruptures 6
    intervertebral disc *see* intervertebral
        disc
    intervertebral foramina 8, 12
    lateral flexion 12
        with rotation 98
    ligament *see* ligament
    muscle contraction effect on 8,
        9(*figs*)
    muscles 8–9, 120
    neural arch 4
    rotation 12
        with lateral flexion 98

wedge, use of during:
    driving 90–1
    re-education of sitting posture 88–9
    sitting 80–1
wedge compression of vertebral
        body 42
writing posture, child/teenager 136,
        140
writing slope, use of 82, 140–1

yoga 130